T0366703

HIV AND AIDS IN AFRICA

HIV AND AIDS IN AFRICA

Douglas Webb

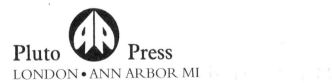

Pluto Press
LONDON • ANN ARBOR MI

David Philip
CAPE TOWN

University of Natal Press
PIETERMARITZBURG

First published 1997 by PLUTO PRESS
345 Archway Road, London N6 5AA
and in Southern Africa by
David Philip Publishers (Pty) Ltd,
208 Werdmuller Centre, Claremont
and University of Natal Press
Private Bag X01, Scottsville 3209,
South Africa

ISBN 9780745311241 (pbk) Pluto Press
ISBN 0745311245 (pbk) Pluto Press
ISBN 9780864863416 (pbk) David Philip & University of Natal Press
ISBN 0864863411 (pbk) David Philip & University of Natal Press

A catalogue record for this book is available from the British Library
and the Library of Congress

Designed, typeset and produced for Pluto Press by
Chase Production Services, Chadlington, OX7 3LN
Printed on Demand by Antony Rowe Ltd, Eastbourne

Contents

List of Figures

List of Tables

Acknowledgements

Many people have played a part in this work, and through the process of travelling many have assisted in some way and since been forgotten. Their help has still been invaluable. For those warranting a mention, I extend my sincere thanks for their enthusiasm, advice, practical assistance and overall their belief in the work. Being pushed all the way by people who wished they had more time to help has been a constant inspiration.

In South Africa: Malcolm Steinberg, Rob Fincham, Pat Liebertrau and all then at the Institute of Natural Resources in Pietermaritzburg, Rose Smart, Greg Wood, Michael Worsnip, Dudu Shoba, Geoff McCarthy, Eleanor Preston-Whyte, Debbie Trompe and all involved with Dramaide, Quarraisha Abdool Karim, Neethea Naidoo, Mary Crewe, Steve Tollman, Joan Cameron, Tennyson Lee, Max Price, James McIntyre, Mpho and Salus in Moloro, Shirley Ngwenya, Prakash in the computer centre in Pietermaritzburg, Alan Whiteside, Jonathan Stadler, Chris Rogerson, Keiran Ndawo, Izak Fourie, Alan and Jill Pugh and all at Tintswalo, Judith Head, Ron Ballard, and special thanks to Alan and Claire Fleming, for being friends as well as colleagues.

In Namibia: Chris Tapscott, Bruce Frayne, Sakira Nghikembua, Andy Botelle, Martin Schabler and all at NISER, Christo Bester, Salmi Imbondi and all in Oshakati State Hospital, Martha Kamati, Maija Palander, Gail Super, Annie Symonds, Mandy Baas, Michaela Figeira, Tim Claydon, Rodney and Wabei Hobson and Sister Kunigunde in Okatana. Many thanks also go to Fiona Farrell for her patience and Leo O'Keefe in Lusaka for his comments and suggestions.

In England: the Economic and Social Research Council who funded the research, Anthony Zwi, Tony Barnett, Piers Blaikie, Mark McCarthy, Sue Lucas, Mark Lloyd, Justin Jacyno, Tim Unwin, Felix Driver, Adrian Walkling, Sarah Gowers, Jeremy Makin, David Simon for his invaluable guidance and supervision, and the staff at Royal Holloway for their constant interest as well as their admirable tolerance.

Preface

The spread of HIV/AIDS across the globe is now unfortunately a familiar story. The changing structure of populations will have untold effects on the way societies organise and reproduce themselves. The documentation of this change from one situation to another, from the pre-AIDS to the post-AIDS era, is essential to allow us to see the future and plan for it to the best of our abilities with our limited resources. In southern Africa, a region emerging from 30 years of civil war and mass political and social instability, this transition will be painful. Those meant to be leading the reconstruction process are coughing and dying, with their children growing up in a situation characterised by poverty, uncertainty and a new donor-driven colonialism. The context of life in the new southern Africa is increasingly one of HIV/AIDS, and we need to know what this actually means, not just as an academic exercise, but as an effort in preventing social and economic breakdown.

Since the recognition of a new disease in the United States in 1981 the search for a cure has proved fruitless and one is unlikely to be found and made widely available before the end of this century. By that time the disease will have claimed the lives of millions of people. The failure of the medical community to provide an answer to the HIV/AIDS issue has placed an unprecedented emphasis on the social sciences to address what is now the most studied disease in history. Still, success in combating the disease evades us, and the list of unanswered questions regarding the socio-behavioural dynamics of HIV/AIDS continues to grow, with increasing recognition of the inherent complexity of the epidemic. The importance of understanding the complex dynamics of the epidemic is often overlooked, to the detriment of the formulation of appropriate prevention programmes. The need for this understanding is the core theme of this book.

In Lusaka, where I now live and work, the impact of HIV/AIDS is evident all around. Absenteeism of colleagues and friends from work for funerals is now so regular as to be expected. Leopard's Hill Cemetery on the outskirts of the city is growing at a phenomenal rate. The road leading to it from the city's main hospital is occupied daily by a series of funeral processions: trucks, buses and open *bakkies* full of singing women. The only booming industry in eastern Lusaka near the cemetery is the small scale production of headstones (plain pieces of slate) and the sale of plastic wreaths, which are then collected from the gravesides and resold. Death is an industry in Lusaka and emotional immunity to the death toll is necessary to continue working in a country where between 20 and 30 per cent of adults are HIV-positive, and thus destined to die within the next ten years or so. Hard, reliable information surrounding the epidemic is in short supply. Despite my recent collation of over 200 research articles and documents on HIV/AIDS in Zambia for a Ministry of Health/UNICEF publication (Webb, 1996a), our knowledge of the situation in this country remains very incomplete. The thirst for this information is striking, and underlies my desire to see this work available to people who need it. Throughout the research period in South Africa and Namibia I was struck by the sense of urgency and interest by colleagues in the results of the work – people who had every inclination but possibly not the time nor the frame of mind to do small scale research in their own workplace and community.

As a consequence, this is not designed to be a text book. The aim is to present a study of the epidemic in a way which is accessible to all. To those involved in fighting the epidemic in the field, this book is meant to provide some insights into the way the epidemic moves around them by understanding the social, economic and behavioural processes involved in the spread of HIV. Many of the topics discussed will be familiar at a superficial level, but the holistic approach taken in looking at the social epidemiology of HIV is rarely attempted. The complexity of HIV spread is not to be underestimated. Many of the reasons for the failure of prevention programmes to date lie in this over-simplification, in reducing the epidemic to medical or health terms, to talk of HIV/AIDS as if socioeconomic processes were merely incidental. The application of social theory in my analysis has surprised health workers here in Zambia and in South Africa, but the benefit to their understanding is obvious. This attempt to open the eyes of HIV/AIDS workers, health and development workers, NGO members, policy makers and researchers to new ways of looking at the epidemic requires much evidence to support it. I therefore make no apology for the amount of empirical data in this book, some of which has been published elsewhere. In essence the data is the backbone of the argument that an holistic approach to prevention planning is essential to achieve success, and the recognition of the limitations of interventions. The empirical data, gathered in South Africa and Namibia during 1992 and 1993, document the social responses to HIV/AIDS at a turbulent time in the history of the region. My experiences in Zambia have only added to my conviction that the important questions are yet to be taken seriously. How does structural change affect behaviour patterns and the way people think about disease? Why is knowledge not translated into widespread behaviour change? The answers lie in the communities and lives of the people with whom we work. This book aims to show how these thoughts, actions and lives can be untangled to reveal the real issues involved in the epidemic: poverty, fatalism, uncertainty, violence and the lack of access to crucial services. The information and knowledge we need to address the epidemic in a more constructive way are therefore localised, and generalisations negate the reality of the great diversity and variety in the way people react to this unprecedented situation. The ultimate answer of prevention is yet to be found but evidence points to the need to reconceptualise the whole idea of prevention into a long term intervention approach, with awkward political questions raised regarding resources, human rights and empowerment. While documenting the present situation we can provide insights for future activity and the ways in which hope can be mobilised and the epidemic eventually overcome. Great efforts were mobilised to overcome smallpox, and it seems that the days of leprosy and even polio are numbered. I produce the work with the aim that insight can and will inform future thinking and intervention. The lives of millions depend on this foresight, and we must not shirk the enormous challenge that faces us all.

*Dedicated to those who are affected,
and those who will be affected
by HIV/AIDS in southern Africa.*

1 The HIV/AIDS Epidemic in Southern Africa

The emergence of the disease now known as acquired immune deficiency syndrome (AIDS) in the early 1980s coincided with a period of social transition in southern Africa, characterised by rapid political and structural change. Why this disease has captured the attention of academics, politicians, business organisations and the general public at large is related to its potential for massive social and economic disturbance. This theme of adverse change, manifested through the use of a range of terms such as 'impact' (Fleming et al., 1988), 'jeopardy' (Panos, 1990) and 'crisis' (Masters et al., 1988) is recognised at a global scale and seen to be inexorable in its progression. The Joint United Nations Programme on HIV/AIDS (UNAIDS) estimates that there have been around 7.7 million AIDS cases by July 1996, with around 22 million people living with HIV world-wide, 90 per cent of whom are in the developing world.[1] The Global AIDS Policy Coalition (GAPC), however, put the number at over 30 million in early 1996, representing a current infection rate of 13,000 per day.[2] Projections for the number of infections by the end of the decade are between 30–40 million (World Health Organization) and 70 million (GAPC).

The disease, or more correctly the syndrome, has been portrayed as having taken on a character of malicious intent, with its own destructive teleology, becoming, in the minds of some observers, a 'killer disease' (Agadzi, 1990), a 'slow plague' (Gould, 1993) and a 'misery seeking missile' (Sabatier, 1988). The syndrome has now become the most studied disease in history and has spawned a host of journals, books and newsletters devoted to its study and monitoring. The study of the geography of the epidemic, through its regional variations and implications for social and economic systems, has only grown as a sub-discipline in the last few years, long after it was realised that AIDS was more than simply a medical phenomenon. Regional study of the disease has focused primarily on Africa, the continent most affected by the human immuno-deficiency virus (HIV), containing an estimated 60 per cent of global infections, although attention is now being paid to Asia in more recent years. In sub-Saharan Africa an estimated 13.3 million adults are HIV-infected.[3] Research into the impact of the disease is still increasing and becoming more multidisciplinary in nature, as the prospect of a cure for AIDS, or a vaccine against HIV, remains remote.

Southern Africa has been under-studied as an area of interest in relation to the social epidemiology of the pandemic. This is especially the case with South Africa, while the literature on Namibia is almost non-existent.[4] At the 1996 International Conference on Aids held in Vancouver, not one paper even mentioned Namibia. Most research in Africa has centred on various 'hot spots', notably Abidjan (Côte d'Ivoire), Kinshasa (Zaire), Nairobi (Kenya), Rakai District (Uganda), Tanzania, Kigali (Rwanda) and to a lesser extent The Gambia. In southern Africa, research has been concentrated mainly in Lusaka, Harare, Johannesburg and Durban, but hitherto with less intensity and funding than work in central and east Africa (Akeroyd, 1994). As a result, the extrapolation of results to a national or even regional scale has been the implicit norm. However, in a continent with 52 countries and much cultural and social diversity, this extrapolation has been misleading and possibly futile, as the geography of the epidemic has proved to be extremely complex, with great spatial diversity in both the epidemiology of HIV and the reported effects of the epidemic. This book explores this diversity and its implications for understanding the epidemic at a local scale.

In South Africa, work on the social aspects of the AIDS epidemic has been conducted almost exclusively by non-geographers, and medical geography as a sub-discipline in South Africa has mostly concentrated on the spatial distribution of health services. As Dauskardt (1992, p. 208) noted, 'the spatial diffusion of many diseases, such as AIDS, remains uncharted'. This book aims to provide a social geography of the epidemic in southern Africa, with specific reference to South Africa and Namibia. The focus, though, is beyond the simply spatial aspects, and concentrates on the crucial issues of community responses to the epidemic, while attempting to understand the complex mechanisms within the social epidemiology (social relationships determining the shape of the epidemic) of HIV/AIDS, and outline some implications for AIDS prevention initiatives. These initiatives have had very little impact on the course of the epidemic to date, and the reasons behind this failure need exploring. The complexities of the obstacles facing AIDS prevention strategies are still not clearly understood, and this book aims to examine certain aspects of this resistance, which prove to be manifest at all socio-geographic scales, from the individual through to the structural.

The Biology of HIV/AIDS [5]

The cause of AIDS, identified in 1983, is a retrovirus which, since 1986, has been known as the human immuno-deficiency virus (HIV). The retrovirus group includes the simian immuno-deficiency virus (SIV) and the human T-cell lymphotropic virus (HTLV) which was identified in 1980. The virus, once within the blood stream, targets the CD4 T-lymphocyte cells, which constitute a vital component in the immune system, as they coordinate antibody production and all immune responses. HIV viral RNA is transcribed to DNA within the T-cell cytoplasm. The viral DNA is then incorporated into the host's nuclear DNA. Replication of the cell results also in viral replication, possibly concentrated within the lymph nodes.[6] Drugs such as azidothymidine (AZT) slow down this replication process, but ultimately do not prevent it and the onset of AIDS is merely delayed. Controversy still surrounds the effectiveness of AZT in preventing the onset of AIDS, but hope is now being expressed of the role of AZT, along with vitamin A supplementation, in preventing mother to child (perinatal) transmission of HIV. The greatest hope in the short term will be the continued trial of protease inhibitors, which are purported to reduce HIV replication to the extent that it is 'undetectable' in the body. The body's production of antibodies to HIV takes place in the weeks following infection (the phase of seroconversion), where approximately half of those infected suffer limited flu-like symptoms. This phase is vital in the detection of the virus in the blood stream, and is discussed in relation to screening. The compromising of the immune system occurs when a proportion of the T-cells are gradually destroyed, so affecting immune responses, but this process is by no means understood. This process has trigger factors that are currently unspecified, which has led some scientists to believe that HIV is not the sole cause of AIDS. The weight of evidence for the HIV-AIDS link is now so overwhelming, however, that few scientists doubt it, although the issue raised considerable furore during 1993–94 when the sceptics were given enormous media exposure. The whole process of HIV related acquired immune deficiency can take over a decade in many individuals, and many children infected with HIV have entered mid-teenage and remained asymptomatic, such as a 15-year-old girl in the United States who has become pregnant despite being HIV-positive since birth. But these cases are exceptions, and the onset of AIDS is usually before a decade after infection. Because of this deterioration process, Max Essex has paraphrased AIDS as the 'Acquired Irreversible Destruction of the immune System'.

In environments where there is a high background level of pathogens, such as in many developing countries, this process of immune deficiency is believed to be considerably shorter than the average of ten years seen in the West, averaging around six years between HIV infection and death. The compromised immune system fails to halt the development of opportunistic infections, 26 of which have been classified by the WHO to date, although the precise definition of AIDS is under constant review.[7] An increasingly common symptom of AIDS in southern Africa is Kaposi's sarcoma, a previously little-understood form of cancer, the cause of which has now been confirmed as a sexually transmitted virus of the herpes family. In parts of Zambia, for example, field workers now consider this one of the most common manifestations, having been virtually unknown only a decade ago. In the early 1980s a new aggressive form of Kaposi's sarcoma alerted doctors in Lusaka that a new disease was endemic in Zambia, and the link with HIV (or HTLV-III as it was then known) was made soon after. The most common opportunistic infections in Africa are tuberculosis (TB), cryptosporidium (gastro-enteritis) and herpes zoster, combined with various oral and skin lesions such as candidiasis and pharyngitis. These conditions, which can combine to cause full-blown AIDS, are themselves regarded as AIDS-related complexes (ARCs) in the presence of HIV infection. The period of full-blown AIDS usually lasts no more than two years, with eventual death resulting from the combined impact of the opportunistic infections.

Two types of HIV have been identified, namely HIV-1 and HIV-2. Recent reports of a third type of HIV discovered in the

Cameroon point to the possible existence of many more variants and a high mutation rate. In recent years these variants have been classified further, with varying degrees of transmissability and virulence (Hu *et al.*, 1996). HIV-1 is far more geographically extensive than HIV-2, which is mostly confined to West Africa. The clinical manifestations of AIDS are similar for the two strains, although the onset of immune deficiency appears to be slower with HIV-2. The viruses are both transmitted in the same ways, which involve the mixing of body fluids.[8]

Heterosexual or (male) homosexual intercourse (horizontal transmission). The virus is found in blood, seminal and vaginal fluids. The presence of venereal infection, particularly those which cause ulceration or lesions, such as syphilis and genital ulcer disease (GUD) increase the likelihood of transmission by up to a factor of four (Laga *et al.*, 1991; Robinson *et al.*, 1993). For example, a study in Rwanda found that over 70 per cent of patients with a sexually transmitted disease (STD) were HIV-positive (Piot, 1993). This point is crucial in South Africa, for example, where 15–20 per cent of the sexually active population have a history of STD (Whiteside, 1993), and STD has been shown to be a crucial cofactor in HIV infection amongst miners on the West Rand.[9] In Soweto, HIV-positive women have a positive serology for syphilis of 20 per cent, which is double that for HIV-negative women (McIntyre, 1993). In heterosexual intercourse, transmission is more efficient from the male to the female (Berkley *et al.*, 1990). Homosexual and heterosexual intercourse constitute an estimated 1 per cent and 93 per cent of adult infections in sub-Saharan Africa respectively (Mann *et al.*, 1992).

From mother to child (vertical transmission), causing paediatric AIDS. The WHO estimates that approximately one third of children born to seropositive mothers will themselves be HIV-positive, and separate studies in Africa suggest that vertical transmission occurs in roughly 20–40 per cent of seropositive pregnant women. The causal factors behind perinatal transmission are not fully understood. A child may be infected via the placenta, during passage down the birth canal (intrapartum infection) or through breastfeeding. There is still much debate over the extent to which breast milk can transmit the virus from mother to child, and evidence is conflicting, resulting in policy dilemmas whether to encourage breastfeeding for seropositive mothers or advocate bottle milk use. The estimated benefit of breastfeeding by HIV-1 seropositive mothers may only exceed the risk of vertical transmission during the first 3–7 months, thereafter the risk of HIV-1 infection may exceed the benefits of breastfeeding (Nagelkereke *et al.*, 1995). This conflicts with research in Uganda which found no correlation between the presence of HIV-infection in breast milk or the duration of breastfeeding and the transmission of HIV-1 infection to the child (Guay *et al.*, 1995). Research suggests that transmission seems to be linked to maternal vitamin A deficiency which is possibly related to the adverse effect of HIV infection on ß-carotene absorption and vitamin A synthesis in the liver[10] (Semba *et al.*, 1994; Nduati *et al.*, 1995). Children who are HIV-positive usually die before the age of five, but in Africa some have survived until the age of at least eleven, and I have met one healthy HIV-positive child in Zambia who is nine.

Through infected blood or blood products. Blood infected with HIV can be transfused into a patient if it is not screened for HIV. In the early years of the epidemic, thousands of haemophiliacs in Western Europe and the United States were infected with HIV prior to the introduction of widespread screening. They received concentrated plasma from hundreds of donors, so resulting in a high risk of infection. Blood which contains HIV, but does not contain HIV-antibodies, is in the 'window period' which is a period of up to six months. This HIV infected blood is undetectable, and in South Africa it is estimated that 2.2/100,000 units within the blood supply are HIV infected. This figure is comparable to that in the United States and Italy (Sitas *et al.*, 1994). Infected blood constitutes an estimated 4 per cent of adult infections in sub-Saharan Africa (Mann *et al.*, 1992), although the figure may be as high as 10 per cent in developing countries overall, due to incomplete screening.[11]

Intravenous drug use (IVDU). The sharing of infected needles has accounted for an estimated 7 per cent of infections worldwide (Mann *et al.*, 1992). The extent of IVDU in southern Africa is unknown, but is likely to be on the increase, as South African cities and Lusaka in Zambia in particular are becoming major drug trafficking centres.

Other means of transmission are far less frequent, such as parenteral infection (needle stick injury or re-use of an infected needle in a medical setting) and through the use of infected blades in circumcision rituals, scarification and traditional medicine. Biting insects, such as mosquitoes and bed bugs, are not vectors of the virus. HIV has been detected in human saliva, but this is not responsible for transmission during deep or 'French' kissing.

The actual measurement of 'seroprevalence', or the *proportion of a defined group of people who are carrying HIV at one point in time*, is done using various techniques designed to prove that HIV is present in the blood. The basic method is the detection of antibodies raised against many or select HIV viral antigens. A universally recognised, efficient and relatively cheap test is still being sought. There are four basic types of test, each with its own specific problems:

- *The Immunofluorescence test.* HIV infected T-cells are used as the antigen source, using immunofluorescence for detection. The test is relatively inexpensive and does not require specialised equipment, but a highly trained technician is needed to interpret results.

- *The ELISA (Enzyme-Linked Immuno-Sorbant Assay) test.* This is the most common group of tests, and has been improved considerably since its first use in the mid 1980s. It is easy to use and is commercially available, with results being provided in a couple of hours. The test is highly sensitive to antibodies but this sensitivity does not overcome the problem of the 'window period'. Retesting tends to reduce the margin of error and prevent false positive results and the subsequent (unnecessary) stress of the person tested. Misuse of the testing kit, such as inappropriate storage, can render the test vulnerable to cross-reactive agents, such as malaria parasites, which give false positive results. Refinement of the test has improved its accuracy to within 1 per cent.[12] ELISA positive tests are often confirmed using the Western blot test.

- *The Western blot test (immunoblot).* This detects antibodies directed at specific HIV viral proteins. This is the most widely used confirmatory test, but is very costly at US$20–35 per test, and the user needs a high level of training.

- *The Rapid Field test.* This is for use in the field, allowing the testing of blood directly rather than plasma. Due to its speed and reliance on precise interpretation, this type of test is considered as only an indicator – the margin of error is too high when practitioner mishandling and inadequate training of the user are considered.

A new test is currently being developed to complement tests already available and possibly even to replace them. The new ImmunoDot screening test is very inexpensive at only US$0.25 per test, does not require refrigeration, and provides results within 20 minutes. Its eventual use is therefore being widely advocated for research and monitoring in rural Africa.[13] Researchers in Mexico have announced the first cost-efficient HIV detection method using saliva. The method is apparently almost 100 per cent sensitive, as well as being faster and less expensive than traditional blood tests.[14] This is obviously a field which will develop rapidly over the next few years.

Age and Gender Differentials in HIV Infection

As HIV is sexually transmitted, the infection profile differs according to age group. Amongst females, the patterns found in Botswana (Figure 1.1) and South Africa (Figure 1.2) are typical for sub-Saharan Africa. HIV prevalence peaks in females in the 20–24 age bracket, indicating that females in teenage and the early twenties are most at risk of infection. The younger age groups are most vulnerable due to a myriad of reasons: economic, sociological and physiological. An exploration of these themes forms a large part of this book.

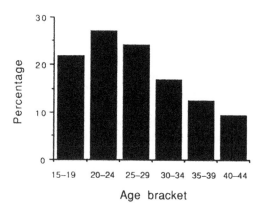

Figure 1.1. HIV prevalence amongst pregnant women by age group, Botswana, 1992–93

Source: National AIDS Control Programme, Ministry of Health, Second HIV Sentinel Surveillance in Botswana, Gaborone, June 1993.

An emerging trend in sub-Saharan Africa is the divergence
of male and female infection rates. In some parts of Africa,
especially in central and eastern regions, women seem more
vulnerable than men, with the ratio approximately 1:1.5. This
gender differential is related to both physiological and cultural
reasons. Studies in Western Europe and the United States have
demonstrated that male to female transmission of the virus is
more likely than female to male transmission per intercourse.
This is mostly due to the physiology of the vaginal wall, the
vulnerability of dendritic cells to the entrance of the virus, and
the longer length of time which the vaginal mucosa is exposed
to genital secretions compared to the male.

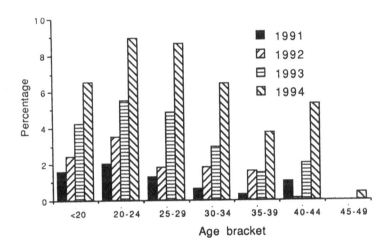

Figure 1.2. HIV prevalence amongst pregnant women by age
group, South Africa, 1991–94
Source: Department of Health, *Epidemiological Comments*, vol. 22, no. 5, May
1995.

The vulnerability of the vaginal epithelium may also be
compounded by the use of oral contraceptives and certain sper-
micide creams, often used by prostitutes (Simenson *et al.*,
1990).[15] In Durban, the male:female ratio of HIV infection
among STD clinic attenders was 1:1.5 (O'Farrell and Windsor,
1989), while a separate study in Natal found an infection ratio
of 1.3:2 (Abdool Karim *et al.*, 1992). Across South Africa as a
whole, the ratio is estimated to be approximately 0.73:1 (*Epi-*

demiological Comments, 1994). This divergence in infection rates has been translated into differential AIDS case rates, as Figure 1.3 demonstrates.

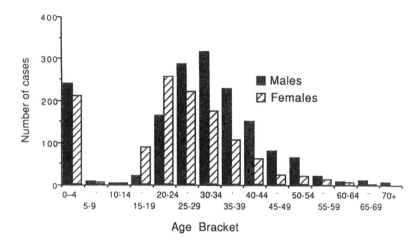

Figure 1.3. Age and sex distribution of reported AIDS cases in South Africa, as at February 1994
Source: *Epidemiological Comments*, vol. 21, no. 2, 1994, p. 40.

The AIDS case rate peaks in the 20–24 age cohort in females and the 30–34 cohort for males. This age difference is accounted for by patterns of sexual behaviour which are characterised by older men having relations with younger women (Chapter 4). This age/sex profile is similar to that for other areas of Africa, indicating that common processes are operating (Mann *et al.*, 1992, pp. 76–8). The low case rates in the 5–14 year old age range point to this group being the 'window of hope' generation, and stresses the need to focus prevention efforts within this age band. This is discussed in detail in Chapter 6.

Patterns of HIV Spread

The different transmission methods described above have their own geography, and on a global scale three epidemiological patterns were defined in 1986–87 (Chin and Mann, 1988), which have since been modified into the categorisation of ten

'Geographic Areas of Affinity', each characterised by a specific epidemiological profile of transmission types, along with similar societal contexts. Sub-Saharan Africa, for example, is one such Area.

- *Pattern I* spread is primarily through homosexual activity and IVDU. Males dominate amongst those infected, with a male to female infection ratio of about 10–15:1. Regions with Pattern I spread are the United States, Western Europe and Australia. The early stages of the epidemic in South Africa were characterised by this pattern.

- *Pattern II* spread is primarily through heterosexual intercourse with the male to female ratio at roughly 1:1. Due to vertical transmission, Pattern II spread is also characterised by an increasing incidence of paediatric AIDS. Regions affected by Pattern II spread are those of sub-Saharan Africa, and increasingly, Latin America, along with parts of South America and India. Over time, it is assumed that Pattern II takes over from Pattern I as the principal mode in terms of the number of cases, if behavioural change is minimal and HIV begins to spread through the heterosexual population. A clear documentation of a country where this has happened has not been produced, however, due to the time lag between the spread of the virus from the high risk groups to the general population. The determining factor here is the 'reproductive rate' of the virus. For the virus to survive in any population, an infected person must infect at least one other person (May and Anderson, 1987). In some countries, including Britain, the reproductive rate has been low enough[16] so far to delay the widespread movement of the virus from high risk groups to the general 'background' population.

- *Pattern III* In Pattern III regions, the spread of the virus is very minor compared to Pattern I and Pattern II areas. Often infected needles are to blame (as in a children's hospital in Romania) or the virus is contained within a small prostitute population. Obviously the potential is there for a Pattern III area to develop rapidly into a Pattern II area; countries of South East Asia, especially Thailand, with its active sex tourism industry (Usher, 1992), are most at risk.[17] Eastern Europe is also very much at risk, given the taboo nature of sex in some societies. In Russia, for example, homosexual activity was until recently illegal, and this could only have inhibited the effectiveness of education programmes.

In all of the regions where HIV is spreading, it is most predominant in urban areas, with an estimated urban–rural ratio of 3.6:1 in sub-Saharan Africa. The reasons for this geographical differentiation relate to the concentration of high risk behaviour in urban localities, linked to prostitution and multi-partner behaviour, as well as the fact that cities and large towns are often the first entry point of the virus into a country, leading to a 'cascade' diffusion down the urban hierarchy (Smallman-Raynor *et al.*, 1992).

HIV Surveillance

Monitoring the spread of HIV involves testing population subgroups for the presence of the virus. Sentinel sample groups often consist of antenatal clinic attenders, blood donors, STD clinic attenders, hospital in-patients and prostitutes. There is a degree of uncertainty as to the extent of the representativeness of the results in relation to the sexually active population, but antenatal data and blood donors are deemed to be the most accurate proxy indicators. Research from Tanzania indicates that blood donors are actually the most representative of sentinel survey groups, even more so than antenatal clinic attenders, provided that the data are standardised for age, sex and urban/non-urban location (Borgdorff *et al.*, 1993), although caution must still be used in interpreting the results as studies in the same area have indicated. For example, Nyamuryeking'e *et al.* (1993) found that the accuracy of blood donations as indicators of general seroprevalence is not constant through time, so making time series studies necessary. The actual structure of the blood donor group is also vital, as different prevalence will be found according to whether the group consists of school youth (relatively low prevalence according to age cohort), out of school youth (relatively high prevalence by age cohort) or those beyond school age. A separate study, also in Mwanza, Tanzania, found HIV prevalence in blood donors of 1.6 per cent, 4.6 per cent and 10.5 per cent for these three categories respectively (Jacobs *et al.*, 1993). The extrapolation of such data beyond the scale of reference is a common exercise, but is dangerous, given the extreme geographical variability of HIV prevalence.

Figures related to the number of AIDS cases must be treated with extreme caution due to under-reporting, which is unquantifiable and varies according to country and over time. For example, Zimbabwe had officially reported 38,552 AIDS cases to the WHO by December 1994, while Dr Evaristo Marowa in Zimbabwe estimated the figure to be over 60,000 cases by April of that year. Estimates of HIV prevalence vary considerably also; Evaristo put the figure at 750–800,000 people being HIV-positive in Zimbabwe,[18] while sentinel surveillance data indicated an average rate of 20 per cent in 1994 (Gregson and Foster, 1994).

Patterns of HIV Spread in Southern Africa

Southern Africa has Pattern II spread of HIV, with the exception of South Africa, which has both Patterns I and II which are 'socially divorced and progressing together' (Smallman-Raynor et al., 1992, p. 315). This generalisation is becoming increasingly untenable as HIV is now being reported within the white hetero-sexual population. HIV-1 is the dominant strain in the region, even though HIV-2 has been detected in Angola, Mozambique, South Africa and Zimbabwe. Figure 1.4 and Table 1.1 show the estimated HIV prevalence in the sexually active population in southern Africa.

The primary pattern of infection appears to be a southward movement of the virus from the central African AIDS belt (Uganda, Kenya, Rwanda, Burundi and Tanzania) towards and through southern Africa. The regional picture hides many intra-country variations in HIV prevalence, which correspond to urban/rural status (the rural epidemic is generally regarded as being seven years behind the urban epidemics and may stabilise at an urban:rural ratio of around 1.4:1; Caldwell and Caldwell, 1993), proximity to primary road networks, and distance from the central African AIDS belt. The picture is not a simple one, and movements of the virus follow movements of people, implicating the processes of oscillatory migration (both international and internal), movements of refugees and inter-nally displaced people (such as returnees to Namibia and Mozambique[19]) business travel of the elite and frequent, local-ised cross-border movements.

An analysis of the patterns of HIV-1 infection amongst an-tenatal clinic attenders in Zambia and Botswana, for example

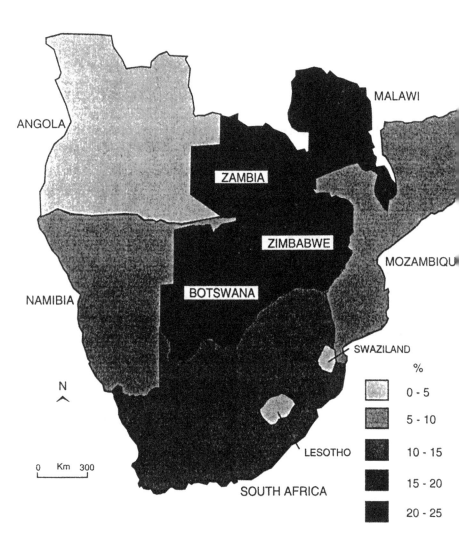

Figure 1.4. Estimated HIV prevalence amongst the sexually active population in southern Africa, 1995
Source: WHO, July 1996; Whiteside, 1995; *SAFAIDS News*, vol. 3, no. 2, June 1995 and vol. 4, no. 1, March 1996.

Table 1.1. HIV/AIDS in southern Africa

Country	Estimated HIV prevalence in the sexually active population (aged 15–59) January 1995 (%)*	Number of reported AIDS cases (last report date)
High prevalence countries		
Botswana	16.5–23	3,110 (Aug 1995)
Zimbabwe	15.9–22	54,744 (Mar 1996)
Zambia	15.8–20	36,894 (Apr 1996)
Malawi	12.3–20	39,989 (Sep 1995)
Low prevalence countries		
Namibia	5.8–8.4	5,101 (Dec 1993)
Tanzania	5.8	45,968 (Jun 1994)
Mozambique	5.1	1,815 (May 1995)
Swaziland	3.4	413 (Feb 1994)
South Africa	2.9–10.4	3,847 (Dec 1994)
Lesotho	2.7	515 (Dec 1994)
Angola	0.9	895 (Mar 1995)

Source: WHO, July 1996; Whiteside, 1995; *SAFAIDS News*, vol. 3, no. 2, June 1995 and vol. 4, no. 1, March 1996.

*   Initial figure represents the 1995 WHO estimate; the second figure represents the estimate from the country's National AIDS Control Programme.

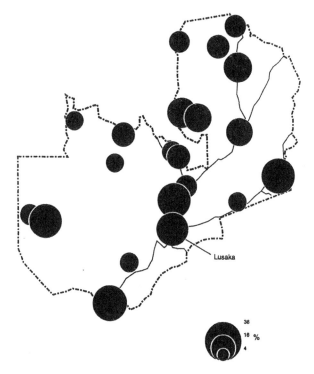

Estimated antenatal HIV prevalence, 1994

Figure 1.5. HIV prevalence amonst antenatal clinic attenders in
Zambia, 1994
Source: Fylkesnes *et al.*, 1995.

(Figures 1.5 and 1.6), demonstrates the extent of these variations. With an estimated 500 new HIV infections per day in
Zambia, and an estimated adult HIV prevalence rate of 10–15
per cent in rural areas and 25–30 per cent in urban, Zambia is
at the heart of the African AIDS belt. Infection rates are expected to peak in urban areas in 1998 at 28 per cent (they have
already stabilised in many urban centres) and in rural areas in
2004 at 22 per cent (Fylkesnes *et al.*, 1995). Infections are concentrated in the urban centres, being highest in Livingstone,
Chipata (both border towns) and the capital, Lusaka, where
prevalences in 1994 averaged around 28 per cent. Lower than
average levels of infection in North Western Province may be
linked to the fact that the ethnic groups in this area, the

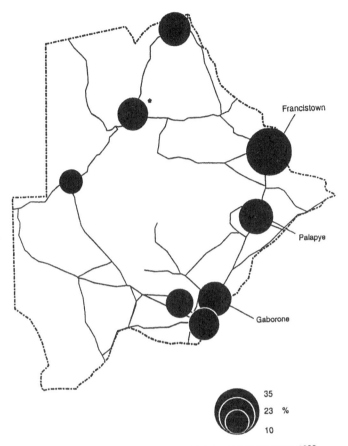

Figure 1.6. Antenatal HIV prevalence in Botswana, 1993
Source: National AIDS Control Programme, Ministry of Health, Second HIV
Sentinel Surveillance in Botswana, June 1993.

N.B. The figure for Maun (*) is an estimate, using the figure for 1992.

Luvale especially, are the only groups in Zambia who consistently circumcise their males (Chapter 2).

A similar spatial distribution, i.e. a rural/urban differential,
is to be found in neighbouring Malawi, with estimated rates of
12.3 per cent and 30.5 per cent respectively.[20]

Within Botswana (Figure 1.6), HIV infection is concen-

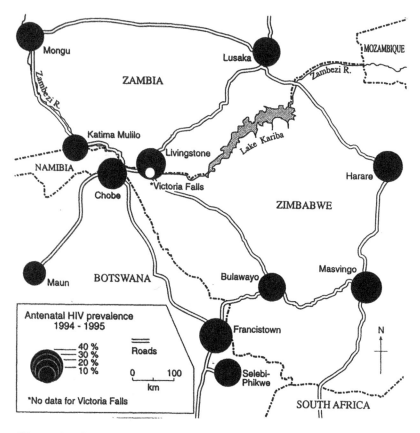

Figure 1.7. Lake Kariba HIV/AIDS nexus
Source:
Botswana – *AIDS Analysis Africa*, vol. 6, no. 3, June 1996.
Zambia – Fylkesnes, 1995.
Zimbabwe – National AIDS Control Programme, Harare.
Namibia – National AIDS Control Programme, 1995.

trated on the eastern side of the country, where population densities are highest. The urban/rural differential is again apparent, with highest rates of infection in Francistown (39.6 per cent), Lobatse (38.9 per cent) and Chobe (37.9 per cent). Overall it is estimated that 23 per cent of the sexually active population (aged 15–49) are seropositive.[21] The high numbers of truckers, migrants and itinerant traders in the country have created an ideal situation for the rapid spread of the virus. A high prevalence in Francistown strongly suggests cross-border movements with nearby Bulawayo in Zimbabwe (Figure 1.7). Francistown attracts many traders (mainly female) from Zambia and Zimbabwe, who are reputedly sexually exploited by police at the border post at Plumtree, who demand sex from women they catch crossing the border illegally. As a local court magistrate commented 'only the ugly ones come to court'.[22] Similarly high prevalences are found in the border town of Livingstone in southern Zambia, where many women make a living by crossing over to Victoria Falls in Zimbabwe, purchasing goods and selling at a marginal profit back in Livingstone. Children are increasingly entering this trade, and young girls are especially vulnerable to sexual exploitation which is closely related to informal sector trading. Interviews with streetgirls in Lusaka for example have shown the high amount of casual sex which takes place between the girls and older men, who prey on their economic vulnerability and destitution.[23]

The situation in Mozambique is not as severe as neighbouring Zimbabwe, Zambia and Malawi but the potential is there for rapid increase in incidence rates. The returnees following the ending of the civil war have come from the above mentioned high prevalence countries. There are an estimated 800,000 HIV-positive people in Mozambique with about 15,000 declared AIDS patients. Antenatal prevalence rates in 1994 within the country ranged from 2.7 per cent in Maputo to 18.1 per cent in Tete. The high rate in Tete can be attributed to the high amount of interaction with Malawi to the east and Zimbabwe to the west, as the main international road runs through this 'Tete corridor'.[24]

HIV/AIDS in Namibia

The HIV/AIDS situation in Namibia is changing rapidly. The first case of AIDS was identified in Namibia in 1986 and there had been 5,101 cases reported by December 1993,[25] with 8,154 known cases of HIV infection by May 1994.[26] The data must be treated with caution as AIDS cases are not differentiated from HIV-positive patients in the figures. HIV-1 is now well established in the small population of 1.4–1.5 million and is spreading at an increasing rate. Antenatal clinic attenders nationwide showed a positivity rate of 4.7 per cent in 1992 (Seidel et al., 1993b), which increased to 8.4 per cent in 1994.

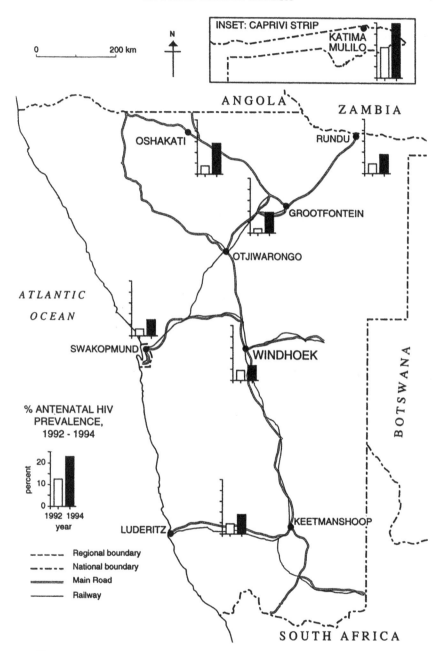

Figure 1.8. Antenatal HIV prevalence in Namibia, 1992–94
Source: see Table 1.2.

Table 1.2. HIV prevalence amongst antenatal clinic attenders in Namibia (%)

Locality	1992	1994
Windhoek	4.2	6.8
Oshakati	3.6	14.2
Katima Mulilo	13.7	24.5
Otjiwarongo/Grootfontein	1.9	8.9
Rundu	4.1	8.4
Swakopmund	2.9	7.3
Keetmanshoop/Luderitz	4.3	8.4
National	4.7	8.4

Source: NACP (1995), Results of National HIV Sero-Survey in Pregnant Women 1994, Press Release, 10 February.

Blood screening was introduced in 1986 and secondary school students are the favoured donor population due to their lower overall seroprevalence (0.6 per cent in 1992). No case of HIV transmission through blood transfusion has been reported to date (Seidel et al., 1993a).

The national figures, however, hide important regional differences, and the epidemiology of HIV within Namibia is surprisingly complex (Webb and Simon, 1993). This complexity is related to an influx of an estimated 45,000 returnees following independence in 1989–90, and a web of migrant labour movements which creates complex sexual networks (Chapter 3).

The probable geographical entry point for the virus is the Caprivi Strip (where positivity rates amongst adults in excess of 2 per cent were reported as early as 1989; Lecatsas et al.,

1989) through cross-border movements to/from Angola and more importantly, Zambia. Interaction with Botswana to the east and South Africa to the south is too low to indicate a substantial influx of the virus, especially as these regions themselves were low prevalence areas in the mid to late 1980s. It is no surprise that the highest prevalence rates at present are in Katima Mulilo (24.5 per cent in 1994). A crucial event was the ending of the war for independence between the South West Africa People's Organisation (SWAPO) and the South African Defence Force (SADF) which finally came to an end in 1989, soon to be followed by Namibian independence in March 1990. Within a period of eight months, 43,387 registered exiles returned to Namibia and, for the most part, resettled in their home locations, the majority of which are in the large northern area formerly known as Owamboland or Owambo (which is now divided into the regions of Omusati, Oshana, Ohangwena and Oshikoto), as well as Caprivi, Kavango and Windhoek (Preston, 1993; Simon and Preston, 1993). These returnees had been in exile mainly in Angola (85.7 per cent of the total) and Zambia (9.2 per cent). Of these returnees, more than 28,000 were aged over 18, and it is reasonable to assume that a significant minority of this group would have been infected during their time in exile. This would represent a sudden influx of the virus into a low prevalence population, so distorting the epidemiology by staggering a smooth progression, depending on the precise movements of the returnee-migrants. Many, ultimately bound for the northern region, opted to return initially to Windhoek, before heading to Owambo where an estimated 33,000 finally resettled. Once returned to Namibia, the repatriates proved to be relatively mobile in their search for work, and were found to be twice as likely to move to seek work than the 'stayers' (Preston, 1993).

Evidence from the northern areas of Namibia suggests that it is this sub-group which is, in part, shaping the early stages of HIV epidemiology in Namibia. If estimates are anywhere near correct regarding HIV prevalence in Angola, approximately 4,000 HIV-infected individuals would have re-entered Owambo during 1989–90, so giving an estimated HIV prevalence of 1.5 per cent of adults in mid 1991, out of a population of 520,000 in Owambo. Official statistics from the Ministry of Health and Social Services (Finckenstein, 1990) placed the cumulative number of AIDS cases in September 1989 at 152,

17 (11 per cent) of which were assumed to have been acquired outside Namibia. As repatriation was still continuing at this time, these 17 infections were probably acquired through cross-border movements, possibly related to trade, but were likely to be unrelated to the repatriation movements. Notably also, 53 per cent of all reported cases were from Caprivi, followed by the Central Region, centred on Windhoek (20 per cent) and Owamboland (8 per cent). Note, though, that these figures relate to AIDS cases rather than to HIV infection. In other words, these figures are still compatible with the claim that repatriation may have introduced 5,600 infected individuals back into the country. A report from April 1993 confirms the sudden rise in AIDS deaths and reported HIV infections. It claims that a total of 51 per cent of the 4,140 HIV cases recorded in Namibia since 1986 were reported in 1992 alone. Of the deaths from AIDS in 1992, 60 per cent occurred in the north-west region (encompassing former Owambo and Kaokoland).[27] In Oshakati in 1994 HIV prevalence rates amongst the sexually active population were about 14.2 per cent. This north-western region is discussed in more detail in Chapters 3, 4 and 5, and gives valuable pointers towards understanding localised HIV epidemiology.

The Geographical Progression of HIV in South Africa

The first case of AIDS in South Africa was reported in 1982 in a white homosexual who contracted the virus while in California. The subsequent Pattern I epidemic was overwhelmingly amongst whites and geographically concentrated in the PWV (Pretoria-Witwatersrand-Vereeniging nexus, now known as Gauteng), Cape Town and Durban. The Pattern II epidemic first emerged in the mid 1980s, but AIDS deaths were predominantly Pattern I type throughout the decade. By 1988, for example, 75 per cent of the 166 reported AIDS deaths had occurred among white male homosexuals (Schoub et al., 1989). The emergence of HIV in the black population was initially concentrated in the PWV area, possibly due to the fact that this area is the centre of the mining industry and thus the focal point for the introduction of the virus by migrant mine workers from the central African AIDS belt (Smallman-Raynor et al., 1992, p. 323).

The annual national HIV surveys of antenatal clinic attenders, compiled by the former Department of National Health

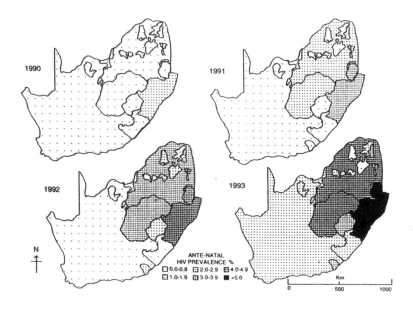

Figure 1.9. The geographical progression of HIV in South Africa, 1990–93

Source: *Epidemiological Comments*, 1994: Webb, D. (1994) Modelling the emerging geography of HIV, *AIDS Analysis Africa*, vol. 4, no. 4, pp. 14–15.

and Population Development, provides a picture of the emerging geography of the HIV epidemic in South Africa (Figure 1.9). For the October–November 1993 survey, blood from 16,207 women was tested (excluding Boputhatswana, which had its own surveillance system until April 1994). It must be noted that those tested in urban areas within each region form a disproportionately large section of the total sample compared to women from rural areas. This bias may cause the overestimation of the true prevalence rate across a whole region. The extent of this bias is unfortunately impossible to quantify exactly. As in neighbouring countries, the 20–24 age group is the most affected. In 1995, 10.4 per cent of antenatal clinic attenders were HIV-positive. The data represent a proxy indicator of the HIV prevalence amongst the sexually active population, but must be viewed with some caution, as the male to female ratio of infection is in the region of 0.73:1. The data also extrapolate a single figure of prevalence across a whole region, so masking the differences related to urban or rural status, or proximity to main roads, which have proved to be major factors in other areas of Africa. In the Transvaal, for example, infection is concentrated on the Witwatersrand, with an urban/rural infection ratio of 2.7:1, according to figures from the Johannesburg City Health Department (*Epidemiological Comments*, 1994). Urban antenatal clinic attenders in Johannesburg recorded a rate of over 7 per cent in September 1993, while a rural area in the eastern Transvaal (Tintswalo Hospital, Mhala, Gazankulu)

Table 1.3. HIV seroprevalence amongst antenatal clinic attenders in South Africa (%)

Province	1990	1991	1992	1993	1994	1995
Western Cape					1.2	1.7
Eastern Cape					4.6	6.0
Northern Cape					1.8	5.3
Free State	0.6	1.5	2.9	4.1	9.2	11.0
Kwazulu/Natal	1.6	2.9	4.8	9.6	14.4	18.2
Mpumalanga					12.2	16.2
Nortern Province					3.0	4.9
Gauteng					6.4	12.0
North West					6.7	8.3
South Africa	0.8	1.4	2.4	4.3	7.6	10.4

Source: Department of Health (1995), *Epidemiological Comments*, vol. 22, no. 5, Department of Health, August 1996.

recorded a rate of below 3 per cent. This urban bias is also demonstrated in the fact that most of the AIDS deaths in the Transvaal occurred in the Central region; by December 1993, there were 821 cumulative reported deaths in the Central Transvaal, with only 86 in the three other Transvaal regions (excluding the former homelands).

Despite the imprecise geographical definition of the data, which also vary according to the year (for instance, in 1990 data were unavailable for most of the former homelands), a broad picture of the regional trends can be drawn (Figure 1.8). The overall pattern in South Africa is one of a movement of the virus south-westwards, with the highest concentrations in Kwazulu/Natal, which recorded an antenatal prevalence of 18.2 per cent in 1995, a figure almost double that of the neighbouring Free State (11.0 per cent). The area of lowest prevalence has consistently been the Cape region, with an increase from 0.2 per cent in 1990 to 1.3 per cent in 1993. This represented a difference in infection rate of a factor of over seven between Kwazulu/Natal and the Cape in 1993, and a gap of approximately four years between the regions in terms of epidemiological progression. In 1995, the infection rate difference between the Cape provinces (average 4.3 per cent) and Kwazulu/Natal had dropped to a factor of four, implying a slow down in the infection rate increase in Kwazulu/Natal. This same time gap is apparent between Kwazulu/Natal and areas of the former northern Transvaal, including the former homelands of Lebowa, Venda and KwaNdebele. This suggests that there is also a northward movement of the virus from the Gauteng into the northern parts of the country, involving migrant labourers in particular; a group which has been shown to be of considerable importance in the epidemic in the Kwazulu/Natal region.

Comparing data from the 1994 and 1995 sentinel surveillance with previous surveys is complicated by the changes in provincial boundaries. Kwazulu/Natal remains the hardest hit area (18.2 per cent), followed by Mpumalanga (16.2 per cent; Table 1.3). The wide inter-regional variation in prevalence rates could be partly explained by patterns of interaction between different areas. The relatively low estimated prevalence of HIV in the former Transkei in 1993 (1.53 per cent) was only just above that of Venda (1.48 per cent) despite Transkei's close proximity to the highest area of prevalence, Kwazulu/Natal. The high number of migrant labourers in Transkei would suggest that the prevalence rate should be higher than it actually is, but patterns of migration could be an important determining factor. Research has indicated that most *male* migrants from Transkei work in the Transvaal, while female migrants are most likely to work as domestics in urban Kwazulu/Natal, so interaction with Kwazulu/Natal is actually more limited than would be expected, especially as regards male migrants (Wakelin, 1983). The most likely infection route into Transkei was therefore from the areas immediately to the north: the Orange Free State and the Transvaal, rather than a simple westward movement from Kwazulu/Natal.

The extent of the difference in infection rates, however, suggests that other risk factors, apart from migrant labour, are involved (Chapter 3). An example is male circumcision, which is mostly absent amongst the Zulu of Kwazulu/Natal but is the accepted norm amongst the Xhosa of the former Transkei. A growing body of evidence demonstrates that non-circumcision is an important risk factor in HIV transmission (see Chapter 2). In addition, the truck routes from the northern areas – Gauteng, Zimbabwe and Zambia – terminate at Durban, with more limited traffic heading down to East London, Port Elizabeth and Cape Town where infection rates are lower and where HIV has evidently been slow to penetrate into the urban hinterlands.

Inter- and intra-regional variations in prevalence rates will persist throughout the course of the epidemic, and the real questions relate to the timing of the eventual stabilisation of the prevalence rate(s) in Kwazulu/Natal, the applicability of this region as a model of the future of the epidemic across the rest of the country, and the pattern of the future stabilisation of HIV prevalence rates across South Africa in the 'low risk' groups. These questions are fundamental to policy makers with the difficult task of budgeting for the immense costs of AIDS in the coming years; insight now can prevent mis-allocation of resources in the future. This topic is discussed further in Chapter 6.

Understanding the Social Epidemiology of HIV/AIDS

This book addresses two basic questions which have extremely complex answers:

- What are the factors which have created the pattern of the social epidemiology of HIV/AIDS outlined above?

• Can these factors be modified, overcome or mitigated in the effort to change the future shape of the pandemic?

Both these questions underlie the explorations throughout this book, and reappear continually throughout the analysis. The conceptualisation of the epidemic is discussed in Chapter 2, and also how the epidemic has been viewed over the last decade. It is argued that the epidemic has been considered in narrow terms, and that the epidemic is the outcome of a complex set of interacting systems fundamentally polarised by the 'individual' and the 'environment'. Chapter 3 identifies the macro-determinants of the epidemic, contextualising the responses of governments, institutions and individuals in southern Africa. The argument is made that the ineffectual responses to the epidemic from governments, and, ultimately, from individuals, can be accounted for by the way that the epidemic failed to be prioritised in the face of more pressing structural problems. Chapter IV explores the behavioural context of HIV epidemiology at the community level, attempting to understand the social and economic processes and linkages involved in sexual behaviour and decision making. The sociosexual environment of HIV epidemiology is documented, and the reasons why HIV is spreading so rapidly are discussed. Chapter 5 analyses community responses to the epidemic itself, and the ways in which social constructions of the disease reflect wider sociopolitical trends and how these constructions affect the course of the epidemic. The positive impact of education campaigns are demonstrated but are shown to have limitations, again due to the fact that the epidemic has not been prioritised, as a result of wider structural concerns, such as violence, poverty, drought and prevailing health problems. The concluding chapter discusses the reconceptualisation of AIDS prevention to incorporate both short term interventions with longer term development initiatives, and their chances of success in southern Africa (and indeed in developing areas generally), which is already facing an epidemic which will have severe economic, demographic and social repercussions.

2 Conceptualising HIV Epidemiology: the Action of the Individual or the Consequence of Place?

The complexity of the HIV/AIDS issue in developing countries, in Africa in particular, necessitates a certain degree of conceptualisation in order to define the parameters of the subject and the relative importance of factors involved. This does not necessarily imply the formulation of models as explanatory or predictive devices, more the representation of different variables in relation to one another. The theories relating to HIV/AIDS in terms of its epidemiology and impact on socioeconomic systems are in a state of flux, to the extent that the methodology of abstraction is far from clear and undergoing constant revision.

Early research on AIDS in Africa considered the context in bio-anthropological terms, examining the cultural variables in any given context, seeking out 'deviance' within 'African' sexuality to provide a quick and 'simple' explanation for the Pattern II (heterosexual) spread on the continent (Chapter 1). The dangers inherent in this 'armchair anthropology' with its racist undertones, have been well documented and anthropologists as well as other researchers found themselves at the centre of a sudden polemical whirlwind that centred on 'African' sexual practices, which supposedly contextualised the epidemic in an explanatory way. As North America and Western Europe were experiencing Pattern I type spread in the mid 1980s, the different pattern(s) seen in Africa led to exploratory accounts of imputed African sexual culture, resulting in a self-defeating closure of research opportunities for Western academics. Epidemiological reports of initial AIDS cases in Zaire, for example, were worded in a way that reinforced cultural and gender stereotypes of assumed black, sexual (and female) immorality in supposed Western terms. At the same time the bio-medical commentators with an interest in 'African AIDS' sought to overlook the vagaries of cultures in pursuit of the universal, and in doing so have created an increasingly disputed 'narration of the real', which is diametrically opposed to the emphasis placed by anthropologists on cultural variability, which is to be expected and essential for the maintenance of community identity. The rich variety of cultures to be found in Zambia (there are 72 ethnic groups in total), for example, testifies to this heterogeneity. Gross simplifications, without spatial or socio-cultural reference, pervaded the literature. For example, Udvardy (1988, p. 94), hypothesised that 'after the introduction of HIV, seroprevalence rates will be higher in matrilineal than in patrilineal, non stratified societies' relating to differences in gender relations and the greater assumed sexual 'freedom' of females in matrilineal cultures. Much debate, however, still surrounds the influence of culture-specific sexual practices, and this work now concentrates on the potential of various 'traditional' activities to increase the incidence of HIV transmission.

There are some major areas under investigation, notably the incidence of ritual cleansing (also known as widow cleansing and levirate union) and its relationship with HIV transmission. To be purged of the 'evil forces' assumed to have caused the death of a spouse, the widow or widower is 'cleansed' through the act of sexual intercourse with a relative of the deceased. This practice is widespread in many countries in sub-Saharan Africa, notably amongst the Luo of Kenya, Rwanda, Zambia and even in South Africa. With the impact of AIDS the practice is undoubtedly on the decline, in Zambia especially, where the chiefs in the Southern Province have been instrumental in encouraging alternatives to sexual intercourse. The adoption of practices such as jumping over brooms or cows which are lying down, or non-penetrative, close body contact has been rapid and encouraging to those involved in behavioural change programmes. Evidently the symbolism surrounding ritual cleansing is more important than the actual act of intercourse itself. Ardent traditionalists in many areas though still perpetuate the sexual aspects of the practice, and the decline in sexual cleansing may be locally very variable, and in a large part determined by the attitude of opinion leaders such as chiefs and the influence of locally based education programmes.

Other anthropological subjects under scrutiny relate to culture and sexual practice, such as the extent of fidelity in polygamous as opposed to monogamous marriages and the practice of inserting foreign bodies such as rocksalt, herbs and leaves into the vagina to increase sexual pleasure ('dry sex'). Male (non)circumcision has been a subject of increasing interest, as circumcision in males appears to be protective against HIV infection to a certain extent. Large scale studies (reviewed in Moses *et al.*, 1994; Caldwell and Caldwell, 1996) have consistently correlated uncircumcised men with higher rates of HIV infection, and this is no doubt related to the physiology of the foreskin and its tendency to 'trap' HIV beneath it, so facilitating transmission. The foreskin is also a site for genital ulcer diseases such as chancroid, the presence of which facilitates HIV transmission. The act of circumcision, however, must never be viewed as a protective measure, as transmission is dependent on a whole host of physiological and behavioural factors. There is a danger that media reporting of these studies instils a false sense of security amongst circumcised men, who subsequently consider themselves to be immune from infection. Female circumcision and the various forms of female genital mutilation are likely to increase risk of transmission, due to the rupturing of scar tissue and increased vulnerability of the vaginal wall. These recent re-examinations of anthropological factors in the epidemic are being done with more caution and in a more interdisciplinary manner than earlier deterministic studies. Self-reflection on the ethics and reasoning behind such a research methodology led to the broadening of research horizons to include the political and economic structures, and *their* possible influence on HIV epidemiology.

Structural analyses of the 'African AIDS' crisis focus on macro-issues and their impact on HIV epidemiology, highlighting the debt crisis with its concomitant economic restructuring programmes, urbanisation fuelled by exploitation by both rural and urban capital along with misdirected government policies, continuing (and indeed deepening) poverty resulting from unequal trade relations with the first world markets, and overseas ownership of key resources and means of production. The importance of capital is certainly not to be underrated, but its precise role and influence at different scales remains poorly defined. The broad structuralist argument, in a sense, is no more enlightening than the bio-anthropological approach in terms of an explanation for observed patterns of infection, as it implies that a certain set of structural conditions will result in a certain behavioural pattern in any given area. The deterministic nature of both approaches cannot account for the variability found at a local scale, but the point is reiterated that the variables determining HIV epidemiology are not just physiological and psychological, but also sociological, economic, and political and always rooted in historical contexts. Conceptually, the identification of three areas of study: the cultural environment, the political economy and the humanist 'life worlds' of individuals can be identified from the literature. The interaction of these three conceptual domains can be represented as a recursive relationship which changes through space and time (Figure 2.1). In simpler terms, behavioural patterns have multilayered determinants, with culture, individual action and sociopolitical factors having differing degrees of importance on the spread of disease at different places at different times. The study of the social epidemiology of HIV/AIDS is the study of this complex interrelationship.

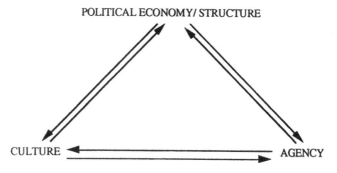

Figure 2.1. Conceptualisation of the study themes within HIV epidemiology (adapted from Schoepf, 1991)

The problem relates to finding a middle-ground providing the terms of reference for an holistic approach, as the knee-jerk reaction of some analysts away from the focus on the culturally determined automaton towards the political economy has been so extreme as to confuse the issue further. In health research generally, the importance of individual behaviour has gradually been eroded, as a quote from McMichael (1993, p. 57) demonstrates (italics my own):

> The important general point – *variations in personal behaviours and local culture aside* – is that the average levels of health risk within populations are largely determined by wider environmental factors, including the stability of ecosystems.

In HIV/AIDS research, the trend has been similar, as individuals are deemed to be hapless victims of HIV infection somehow 'caused' through some sort of environmental determinism. The case is never stated too explicitly, as the result would be analysis devoid of any reference to the capacity of individuals to react differently to a certain set of conditions. This position though remains not only false but dangerous, as individuals are not encouraged to accept responsibility for their behaviour, and can ultimately lead to a sense of irreversible fatalism. The conclusions reached in these analyses lean towards a structural position and have very few implications for localised prevention programmes. For example,

> HIV transmission cannot be curtailed unless the social conditions facilitating its spread – the migrant labour system, vulnerable family relationships, low wage work for women – are transformed. (Jochelson et al., 1991, p. 170)

> The issues which should be addressed are overcrowding and the housing crisis, migrant labour and the collapsing family structure, high unemployment rates and a host of similar politically enforced socioeconomic factors. (Crewe, 1992, p. 16)

> In Africa a review of property distribution laws after divorce may be more important in slowing the spread of the virus than condom distribution.[1]

Over time, a shift in approaches is discernible, with the political economy perspective gaining ground over the behavioural/anthropological approach (Figure 2.2). The shift in emphasis from individual to structure, with the associated implication of causality, has done very little in providing valuable insights into HIV epidemiology and, more importantly, in providing practical guidance to the improvement of prevention programmes working within Africa. The emphasis on structures also runs counter to the current movement in social science epistemology which is re-appraising the role of the individual in relation to life worlds, differential identities, cultural relativism and local constructions of knowledge. Furthermore, the association of causality with macro-structures is tantamount to an admission of 'defeat', and contradicts so much positive work being done on a small scale.

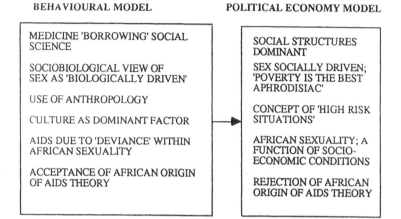

Figure 2.2. Approaches in socioeconomic HIV/AIDS research in Africa, 1985–92 (adapted from Packard and Epstein, 1991)

This position is also claimed for health education in a British context (Winn and Skelton, 1992), but the situation in Africa is seen by some as so desperate as to be 'lost' (Le Fanu, 1991). The general perception of Africa remains a continent engulfed by famine, wars, massacres and ineptitude. Positive movements in health provision and education are often lost in the media fixation for the horrific. Reconstruction and rehabilitation in Rwanda for example is ongoing and involves huge financial and human resources; this is rarely reported. Non-governmental organisations (NGOs), in the face of this overwhelming academic and media pessimism, even periodically issue 'statements of belief' to the effect that large scale behavioural change in relation to AIDS is possible given the provision of adequate resources.[2]

The problem should be redefined in terms of subject matter rather than approach. Any approach which examines some determinants while ignoring others must be avoided, because the determinants act in relation to each other, not as separate entities. Conceptualisation of the situation, if any accuracy is to be maintained, must include all cultural, structural and behavioural factors. An holistic approach, *within a given context*, would thus avoid the problems related to the different approaches. The question would be changed from 'what are the determinants?' to 'how important are the different determinants *in this specific context?*' The partial reconciliation of the two approaches can thus be achieved through the introduction of the concept of the *spatial variability* in the influence of determining variables. 'High risk behaviour'[3] is spatially defined, due, in part, to factors determined by the political economy of the area unit addressed with an intervention. For example, the incidence of prostitution may be higher in one urban street compared to another, relating to the social construction of that particular street, which is itself related to occupational function of the residents, land use type, land value, accessibility, relationship with any legislative bodies, and spatial boundaries inherent in either law or historical association. On a larger scale, social disruption, caused by war or famine, leads to displacement, refugee movement and resettlement of some sort, either in camps or peri-urban environments, where feelings of *anomie* (anonymity and personal vulnerability) may be increased, leading to the breakdown of social norms, not least regarding sexual behaviour. At a national scale, a labour system which encourages the separation of household members (prevalent across southern Africa) would facilitate extramarital sexual contacts at the mine or in the village. This introduction of space, through the study of movement, separation, but also isolation and, more recently, the spatial determinants of *anomie* (Wallace, 1991, 1993), are recent and valuable innovations in the AIDS literature. This aspect of space is discussed later, but suffice it to say in this context that previous models of HIV spread, based on polarised conceptual frameworks, did very little towards providing an adequate template for either explanation or practical intervention in relation to the HIV/AIDS pandemic.

It is difficult to place culture into the concept of 'high risk behaviour' as culture is an aspatial structure in itself, *influencing*, but not determining, marital systems, household structures, sexual mores, circumcision practices and the social use of space. The use and abuse of culture as an explanatory tool is often done by individuals themselves, who can use culture as an excuse for behaviour which may be perceived by some to be immoral. In my experience many individuals allude to cultural heritage without any sound knowledge of that heritage, leading to blatant contradiction. The notion of culture is often used when required as a unavoidable cause of a particular behaviour – in doing so the culture can be debased and misrepresented. The individual allusion to a cultural cause of a behaviour is fallacious; an individual may find him/herself in a situation where HIV infection is a possible outcome of a series of events, be it unprotected intercourse, scarification with an unsterile blade, parenteral infection etc., but this context can be no more than a factor *influencing* behaviour; it does not determine the precise sequence of events and any resultant infection. Behaviour of the individual will vary according to context but it is not determined by it. There is no simple cause-effect link, only a causal relationship based on probability; high risk sexual activity with resulting infection is more likely in context A than in context B.

The context in which HIV/AIDS spreads is thus a subject which can be conceptualised in a number of different ways. This is important in that research questions and intervention design will be very different according to the approach adopted. It is almost impossible to study the socioeconomics of HIV/AIDS in a local setting without having an approach which is theoretical in its framework. The ethics of researching sexual behaviours require that some sort of theoretical framework is adopted, if only to avoid accusations of 'ethnopornography'. An hypothesis is not essential, but must be implicit in the research. As a result, a paradoxical situation is encountered where a theoretical framework is ill-defined and undergoing constant revision, yet, to research effectively, an hypothesis must be incorporated. This is symptomatic of the state of flux within the subject, possibly due to its multidisciplinary and immature character. Locally based studies by clinicians or health workers are often ill-informed and conceptually weak due to this theoretical uncertainty, and many studies which attempt to go any way beyond basic enumeration or prevalence estimates are liable to fall into this trap. This renders the work unusable outside the geographical area of the study and often anecdotal in nature. There is a need for the standardisation of definitions and methodological procedures, as new (and old) epistemologies are reviewed for their efficacy in practical HIV/AIDS research. These issues are taken further in the discussion of methodological considerations towards the end of this chapter.

Alternative Approaches to the HIV Pandemic

This shift of approaches away from the bio-anthropological models, in the light of the failure of medical science to curb the spread of HIV, has necessitated medical sociologists, anthropolo-

gists and geographers to become increasingly involved in intervention programmes and policy formation. The failure to halt the
pandemic is not simply a medical issue, but is integrally linked
in with epistemologies regarding epidemiology and disease causation. As Mayer (1992) has recently pointed out, medical geography would do well to escape from the strait-jacket of the philosophy of logical positivism in which it has been living since its
inception as a sub-discipline. In other words, the 'understanding'
of the epidemiology of a certain disease has been equated with its
description, spatial distribution and explanation, through the
identification of causal relationships. But this definition of causation is founded in positivist philosophy, i.e. the link has to be
observable, verifiable and demonstrable. Alternative epistemologies, though, are no less valid in epidemiology, as the concept of
causation can, and should, be broadened beyond the confines of
positivism. Alternatives to a positivist approach seek to incorporate wider societal structures and their role in determining
health-related behaviour. The terminology differs from author to
author and this is not surprising, given the infancy of the theoretical vocabulary in its association with epidemiology. The
merging of social theory and scientific analysis is in part due to
the failure of the behavioural/bio-medical models in terms of
HIV/AIDS prevention, and is also related to a more advanced
epistemology amongst those seeking explanations for the particular social epidemiology(ies) of HIV/AIDS. As a consequence, ob-
scure terms and technical jargon are liberally sprinkled throughout the new texts without thorough explanation, and this can
lead to the rejection of the texts as valid analyses. An example of
an alternative approach is what is known as *political ecology*:

> The political ecology approach challenges the nature of disease causa-
> tion inherent in the germ theory of disease and the doctrine of
> specific aetiology. Cause, to the political ecologist, lies just as much
> in social structures as it does in microbes. (Mayer, 1992, p. 583)

There are three sub-themes to the political ecology approach:
Realism, Structuration and Marxism. These approaches are almost identical in character when related to epidemiology, as the
explanations they attempt to provide have a similar theoretical
base. The identification of wider structural issues is fundamental
to these epistemologies, and their (inter)relationship with disease
patterns. The concept of causation thus becomes problematic,
with the emphasis shifting from quantitative to qualitative analy-

sis, away from the classical causal definition of 'x can only cause y if x temporally precedes y and that x leads to y in a unidirectional relationship' (Susser, 1987). Within this tradition of positivist analysis, predictability is introduced as an essential concomitant to the identification of causal links. Realism, though ultimately based on thinking first examined by the Scottish philosopher David Hume in the eighteenth century,[4] claims that causation is not necessitated by frequency of association or the replicability of a phenomenon. Two events which are related through repeated observation cannot be rationally justified to have a causal relationship between them. In HIV epidemiology, simplistic causal relationships do not exist as the number of acting variables is too large to define precisely and, by their very nature, many have no quantitative value. Because the epidemic has such a considerable, but again unquantifiable, behavioural aspect, proxy measures of perception, influences on behaviour, knowledge and priorities are needed to produce an estimation of the nature and interaction of the determinants in any one setting. In relation to health risk assessment, Hayes (1992, p. 406) identifies the similar concept fundamental to realism, that of 'closure', or

> the internal structure of the mechanisms that allow something to undergo change (the inherent causal properties or powers of risk relations to lead to specific health outcomes) operate consistently across time and space.

The further a relationship departs from closure, the less the expected empirical regularity of pattern. This has important implications for the understanding of HIV epidemiology, as behavioural and structural determinants vary across time and space. In one village a certain set of factors determines the spread of the virus, but elsewhere different sets are likely to be relevant. The factors which are causally linked (according to conditions of closure) are very limited, if, indeed, any exist at all. For example, the only factor in HIV epidemiology which satisfies the conditions for closure is its actual transmission: the mixing of body fluids of an infected individual with those of an uninfected individual. Even then, transmission and subsequent sero-conversion is dependent on the viral load, the extent of immune suppression in the recipient (in the case of superinfection), lymphocyte density in the genital region, and even possible 'immunity' to infection, which has been purported to be the case with some prostitutes in Nairobi.[5] This relationship, or likelihood of transmission, may have a geography of its own and be linked in with both the incidence of opportunistic infections and STDs. What certainly does vary, and thus have geographical expression, is the other vast set of factors which lead to that incidence of transmission. There is a myriad of reasons why two people engage in unprotected heterosexual intercourse (this being the predominant mode of spread of HIV in Africa). These reasons can be economic, cultural or biological (either procreation, sexual pleasure or rape). For example, the reasons why people engage in sexual relations in a brothel are different from those in a workers' compound, marital bed or teenage party.

As the determinants of the epidemiology of HIV vary across time and space, the exact factors relating to each incidence of transmission are unique. The identification of causal relationships is thus impossible within a positivist framework, and therefore a broader concept of causality is needed. Conditions for closure are never met with the epidemiology of HIV as behaviour and structures are location-specific, and even then the definition of scale is crucial. The way individuals respond to their environment, be it social, cultural or economic, and the general nature of the individual-environment interaction, varies greatly even within single, location-specific population groups:

> It is crucial to approach AIDS as a disease of society, of political economy and culture – both of which can change – rather than simply as a virus spread by individuals. (Schoepf, 1991, p. 759).

The assumption of homogeneity within sexually active groups does not accord with anthropological data which emphasise variation at a local scale (for example, Leavitt, 1991). This aspect of scale must be more carefully considered. The anthropological investigation of the transmission of HIV between two people would yield a complex list of reasons for that particular unprotected sexual act. The addition of externalised perspectives, encompassing structures, would give a more holistic explanation. The set of factors for one individual sex act could be very complex: cultural, economic and behavioural. The extrapolation of this analysis to a societal scale would result in virtually meaningless statements: 'AIDS spreads due to poverty', 'AIDS spreads because of the migrant labour system' and 'AIDS spreads due to a generally immuno-suppressive environment'. The implication of direct causation in each of these statements is very simplistic. Not every individual subjected to poverty has been, or will be, exposed to the virus. Poverty in a certain context may contribute to the spread of the virus but in no way determines it. Even at a micro-scale generalising is problematic, as transmission occurs only in certain locations and at certain times, with different degrees of regularity. Roundy (1987) demonstrated how the transmission of communicable diseases in a rural Ethiopian community varied according to precise location within the community (both social and geographic) and the different degrees of interaction between vectors (both human and non-human) and their hosts. The same is thus true with HIV spread and interventions at the scale of an urban township or compound must be integral to the conditions within that community or communities. The assumption that what will work in one place will necessarily work in another must be avoided, and it is the task of those involved in prevention programmes to understand what particular aspects of a prevention initiative are replicable. So often the success of a programme is dependent on key actors within that community being involved with the design and implementation of the programme. The cooperation and knowledge of local people such as prostitutes, health workers, traditional healers, traditional leaders, educationalists and women's groups is essential.

Structuration Theory

In attempting to understand the social epidemiology of HIV, the analysis concentrates on human behaviour, its motivations and determinants. Appropriate conceptual tools are essential to analyse this behaviour and can be found in structuration theory, which was outlined and refined by the sociologist Anthony Giddens in a long series of publications and debates through the 1970s and 1980s (Giddens, 1984; Cloke *et al.*, 1991). Looking at this particular theory provides a useful set of definitions and concepts which prove to be applicable to understanding the way HIV spreads. The ideas found within structuration theory provide a useful framework for analysing the behaviour of individuals within their social, economic and cultural environments. The problems encountered in the bio-anthropological and structural approaches, namely a polarisation of concentration either on the individual as a cultural entity, or on macro-processes in which individual behaviour is pre-determined, are removed, as the structure-agency analysis encompasses both the individual and environment in a single conceptualisation. Research methodology and approaches are now being modified to become more flexible, in order to address both structures and individuals, such as the work by Caprara *et al.* (1993) on the perception of AIDS in the Côte d'Ivoire. With structuration theory, the concept of causality is also modified. The agency/structure relationship is continuous and recursive, so there is no theoretical starting point for a sequence of causally related events. There is no identifiable temporal division between events – *x* does not precede *y*, *x* interacts with *y* *through* time. In other words, properties inherent in a specific environment do not cause a certain behaviour, but influence behaviour to an extent which is dependent on the individual, and *vice versa*. Some explanation of the terminology of Giddens is essential, along with the simplification of his main tenets. Structuration is useful as a *tool* for understanding HIV epidemiology, as it is a conceptualisation of the influences on behaviour and the motivations for behaviour change. With respect to the spread of HIV, two issues regarding behaviour are under question:

• What are the motivations for sexual activity?

• What are the factors determining HIV transmission within this activity?

Giddens distinguishes between action which is motivated by the individual, *purposive action*, and action which has no motivational cause. This motivation can be conscious, subconscious or unconscious, and Giddens claims that the unconscious element is very important. Individuals (whom he calls agents) assess, rationalise and justify their actions (either to themselves or to others) through the process of *reflexive monitoring*. Accounts for actions will be affected by both the unintended consequences of action, and the *unacknowledged conditions* of actions – these are both collective phenomena, i.e. involving different people such as family, friends etc. The unacknowledged conditions would be elements of the environment which are not part of the conscious decision-making process. Such elements could be the economic structure of an area, cultural norms, gender relations, or the labour profile of any given context, be it the household, community or larger administrative unit. The unintended consequences of action are seen to feed back into the unacknowledged conditions of action, in so doing creating the structures contextualising behaviour, such as the sociological cycle of poverty. People's behaviour regarding sexual activity would be in part related to these un-acknowledged conditions, such as attitudes towards promiscuity, pre-marital sex or polygyny. The extent to which people adhere to these attitudinal influences determines the nature of the influences on future occasions. In other words, some ethnic groups may view pre-marital sex as a normal aspect of adolescent behaviour, while in others there may be much stigma attached, even though the two groups share a common cultural origin. This communal level of acceptability would be interpreted by adolescents, so influencing the extent of pre-marital sex, which would either reinforce the taboo, or conversely, if pre-marital sex over time became a frequent part of behaviour, would cause the acceptability of the activity to be communally and societally reassessed. This reassessment would be unconscious, continuous and take place along age, gender and possibly economic lines as well, leading to a possible contradiction and conflict of opinion within geographically proximal groups, with a resultant heterogeneity of both perception and behaviour. Conflict of opinion in societies of course is extremely common when dealing with sexual matters, and understanding the causes and evolution of such conflicts (such as whether or not sex education in schools is desirable) is extremely useful in trying to address and resolve them. If these conflicts are misunderstood or ignored, an intervention is likely to fail due to resistance from some quarters. Debates over contraception in relation to Catholicism, for example, take many different forms, and interventions must be sensitive to local conditions: the influence and attitude of local opinion leaders, church groups, mission hospital policies and the whims of politicians.

Giddens' next concept relates to the difference between *structures* and *systems of interaction* in the analysis of society. For example, speech, as an action, is time/location specific. Language itself is not locatable in time and space. He identifies structures in terms of a set of rules and resources. Gender relations, as a societal structure, comprise a set of norms and unwritten rules which are constantly modified through female resistance/empowerment or male assertion in a myriad of different ways. These *rules* and the aspect of power associated with these *resources* constrain behaviour both physically, socially and geographically. In real terms, the behaviour of women would be constrained in terms of time budgets, the need to fulfil domestic responsibilities, limited income-earning and travel opportunities, and most importantly in relation to HIV, lack of negotiating skills or influence regarding the incidence of *some* sexual activity, be it protected or otherwise. Research questions which this book addresses relate to the exact nature of these constraints, how they vary spatially and across social groups (by age and income in particular), what feasible intervention strategies exist for reducing these constraints, and how these changes, in turn, relate to women's vulnerability to HIV infection. Giddens himself did not relate the conceptual framework to the issue of gender, but the incorporation of gender within a structuration perspective can help in the understanding of processes such as dependency and empowerment which are explored in Chapter 6.

The next question relates to how these influences on behaviour are maintained and communicated within any given context. Giddens uses the phrase *integration* to conceptualise the link between agents and structures. Integration falls into two categories, *social* integration and *system* integration. Social integration is the daily lives of people, through face to face meetings, speech and direct interaction with others. Telecommunications and transport technology have transformed the time-space of social interaction, so leading to the differentiation of social integration, which is the daily lives of agents, from system integration, which allows for long distance communication, through such institutions as the media and the increased use of information technology. Giddens argues that social integration and system integration come together in particular *locales*. *Regionalisation* is the zoning of time-space in relation to the different forms of interaction, and therefore necessarily occurs at various scales; the home, community, workplace etc. Giddens, though, has not defined a hierarchy of locales and refuses to use the phrases micro and macro; instead insisting on *duality*.

With reference to HIV/AIDS, the importance of these concepts is not immediately apparent, but once the aspect of *scale* is introduced, different determinants of behaviour can be seen to have different spatial influences. For example, AIDS education through the media will have more impact in a locale which has well established links with media institutions such as newspapers, televisions, advertising spaces. Rural populations may have less access to newspapers than urban populations, who would have more complex and thorough accessibility to various information sources. In rural areas, system integration is less developed, and radios may be the only direct link with wider information sources. Most information would come from interaction with other community members, and information generally would be of a more localised nature. Scales of reference are more geographically limited to the immediate environment and community, with only partial contact with distant urban centres (through migrant workers and itinerants), which also function as the main centres of national information dissemination. Firsthand knowledge may be more important in determining behaviour than secondhand information derived through word of mouth reports.

There are various scales to the influences on human behaviour. In terms of the explanation of behaviour, a variety of settings must be considered, with different scales of regionalisation. The precise *locales* are crucial, as individuals would have varying degrees of the influence of structures according to the nature of the locale(s) within which individuals find themselves – the household – the community – the region – the nation state. Is there a gradation of influence with increasing scale? In other words, are people's behaviours more influenced by immediate, social integration, or by contacts through system integration? Do behavioural responses to a locally produced and oriented AIDS education programme differ in nature from the responses to a nationally coordinated programme? Is there a spatial component in the response to AIDS deaths? Would deaths that are spatially disparate have less impact on behaviour change than deaths which were local? These questions have not been explicitly asked in socioeconomic research on HIV/AIDS, but are continually hinted at. An anthropologist, documenting the emergence of the cultural construction of AIDS discourse in the rural Haitian village of Do Kay (Farmer, 1992), noted the extreme place sensitivity of cultural response, which changed dramatically over time. This response was so specific to the village scale that he commented: 'That each of these factors is of changing significance led me, at times, to question the relevance of such fine grained analyses' (p. 299). Such self-reflection comes about upon the realisation that the epidemic, as a socially constructed phenomenon, has distinct and dynamic geographies of its own. Farmer then advocated the use of methodological procedures allied to the techniques of processual ethnography, which 'helps to bring into relief changes in what was important to the people of Do Kay'. His use of a geographical metaphor was apposite in hinting at the need for a new understanding of the epidemic.

The Role of Geographical Research

Where Geography as a discipline would make its contribution in the understanding of the spread of HIV/AIDS has so far been assumed to be little more than in the realm of cartography. Even this particular aspect has been underutilised to date and geographers are only now starting to define their role, relying on grand definitions in the hope of justifying their application to the topic:

> Human geography, for example, attempts to illustrate and account for the spatial variation of human behaviour and the human condition, relying on a composite developed in part from psychology, sociology and anthropology. (Shannon, 1993, p. v)

The spatial aspect of AIDS, however, within its *geography*, is more than simply the mapping of the disease or plotting its spatial representation, although these are very often prerequisites. It involves the *influence of place* on the course of the disease. Assertions to this effect, though, still lack any positive implications and remain at the level of suggestion:

> Spatial representations of comparable seroprevalences, showing time variations and comparisons with other sociodemographic factors may be useful if done rigorously. (Tessier *et al.*, 1993, p. 127)

The sub-discipline of the geography of AIDS is still in its infancy despite recent publications on the subject (Shannon *et al.*, 1991; Barnett and Blaikie, 1992; Gould, 1993; Smallman-Raynor, *et al.*, 1992) and the literature at the present time still calls for more geographically oriented research. Mayer (1983, p. 1213) suggests that geographic studies of disease are valuable for two reasons: 'they suggest possible causal factors in pathogenesis', and 'they serve as indicators of how regions are structured, and of how individuals and groups exist in mutual interaction with the environment'. For example, regarding the spatial representation of AIDS, the question of why HIV prevalence is higher in one place compared to another has three competing explanations:

- There is spatial variation in the prevalence of HIV within the social environment, so with constant behaviour over

space, HIV clustering or aggregation occurs, as the likelihood of infection per sexual act increases or decreases
accordingly.

• There is a geographical variation in risk-taking behaviour,
given a constant likelihood of infection per sexual act, associated with variations in sexual behaviour and/or differences
in condom use/accessibility.

• There is a geographical variation in both the prevalence of
HIV and the extent and type of risk-taking behaviour.

Geographers are able to represent spatial patterns of disease
and in regard to HIV/AIDS, four global patterns have already
been identified (Mann et al., 1992). These patterns, however,
hide inter-regional differences and the aspect of scale again
becomes crucial. In central Africa a boundary to westward HIV
diffusion has been identified which correlates with the political
boundaries between high prevalence countries of the Central
African Republic and Congo, and the currently low prevalence
countries of Chad, Cameroon, Equatorial Guinea and Gabon
(Tessier et al., 1993). There is no ready explanation for this
boundary, but the authors concluded that, 'It is clear that the
HIV epidemic is heterogeneous throughout Africa and follows
different diffusion patterns from one ecosystem to another'
(p. 131). At a localised scale, patterns emerge which are related
to transport infrastructure, economic activity and migration
patterns which in part determine the geographical extent of
infection and the epidemiological regime. Identifying pattern is
one thing, through HIV prevalence or AIDS case rates for
example, but the logistical step to explanation of the pattern is
something very different, and must be done with caution. The
number of interacting variables is so large and the nature of
their interaction so complex, that the misinterpretation of data
(which itself is open to question regarding its reliability and
comprehensiveness) is very possible, and causal links are almost impossible to verify. The task of the researcher in this
context is not to seek causation, but rather to identify relationships, because the role of agency makes the concept of causation obsolete at an individual level. The identified patterns of
disease hint at underlying processes creating that pattern, and
it is this inference which gives medical geography its traditionally positivist *raison d'être*:

Perhaps a task in medical geography which is not yet begun is to develop the rules – the laws – by which cultural, social, economic, environmental and biological factors become translated into the spatial form of disease. (Mayer, 1983, p. 1214)

The shaky philosophical basis for proclaiming causation between two variables in the production of the spatial pattern of HIV, for example, leads to an interpretation based on statistical probability and the identification of risk factors. This probability of infection, given a set behaviour pattern, would vary spatially, and it is this spatial variable which causes the prediction of pattern to be so difficult. Macro-simulation models have to confront this problem through the adoption of certain behavioural assumptions, resulting in probabilistic predictions of the future course of the epidemic (Anderson, 1991; Anderson and May, 1992; Anderson et al., 1991; in South Africa: Doyle, 1993; Southall, 1993; in Zambia: Fylkesnes et al., 1995). This level of uncertainty and variability in the assumptions used to create such models inevitably produces a wide range of possible outcomes, and even then of HIV prevalence or numbers of AIDS cases without specific geographical definition. Their use is thus extremely limited, and are mostly favoured by planners adopting future scenarios for calculating the implications for demographic change (Cross and Whiteside, 1993), urbanisation rates (Whiteside, 1991), costs to insurance firms and various industries, and health services planning (Cross and Whiteside, 1993).

The niche for a geographically oriented approach was implicitly noted by Zwi and Cabral (1991) who called for the identification of 'high risk situations'. The use of the term 'situation' implies the introduction of the spatial variable (although a 'situation' can also be defined in social terms), and overcomes the problems inherent in the use of the terms 'high risk group' (such as truck drivers, prostitutes, soldiers and itinerants), which is exclusionary, and 'high risk behaviour', which sheds no light on the causes of a particular behaviour. Even so, Zwi and Cabral's conceptualisation was part of the trend towards a structural explanation, and in doing so diminished the role of agency. They claim that 'health is far more readily determined by social conditions than by individual behaviour and health services' (p. 47). This is true, but only to a certain extent, as it would certainly not apply in all situations. The 'high risk' situation is characterised by diminished concern about health, increased risk taking, reduced social concern about sexual activity, and the reduced ability to practice safer sex. Willms has expanded the terminology, if not so much the theoretical framework, by analysing 'risk realities' in Zimbabwe (Willms and Sewankambo, 1995).

Clearer attempts at least are being made to link social theory with prevention projects, as there are important implications for concepts of targeting, geographical coverage, peer education and risk reduction through the addressing of local contextual issues such as access to health services and local marketing networks. The important point which is made is that a 'risk' context is recognised as an influence on behaviour. This had been elucidated previously by Baldo and Cabral (1990) in the analysis of the impact of low-intensity wars on risk-taking behaviour regarding sexually transmitted diseases. A full discussion on the issue of causality between structures and individuals in a high risk situation, though, was avoided, because 'these intermediate social processes may be difficult to express mathematically and consequently to allow for the use of common statistical tools to confirm a cause-event relationship' (p. 39). Indeed, the measurement of the influence of place, in terms of its socioeconomic and cultural composition, on health related behaviour has proved to be the stumbling block for many epidemiological analyses. The associated methodology is under constant stringent review, on both practical and philosophical grounds, involving what Gagnon (1992) has termed 'epistemological doubt'. Despite the inherent methodological problems, such analyses are still being conducted, and with results which reinstate the role of environmental influences.

Few analysts have attempted to integrate the aspect of scale into these scientific techniques, with the notable exception of Graham Moon and colleagues in Portsmouth (Duncan *et al.*, 1994). Their use of 'multi-level' analyses attempts to integrate principles inherent within social theory into the modelling of health related behaviour. These models provide the mechanism for the examination of agency within differing structural contexts. Their possible use in the analysis of sexual health behaviour could undermine the validity of the abundance of conceptually flawed studies of sexual health behaviour as regards HIV/AIDS, and lead to the abandoning of the tendency to polarise behaviour and context. Progress has been made by Wallace (1993), who identified crucial structures which he termed as *externalities* that had negative impacts on social networks. Working in Harlem, New York, he identified an all round sense of *anomie* amongst the people living there, and public policies which increased the process of social breakdown, in particular those related to housing. Mathematical modelling of the social networks of internal migration and resource sharing identified thresholds of breakdown:

> Stress on the community ... may, if a critical threshold is exceeded, not only disperse the minority voting block and prevent exercise of political power, but can in fact utterly dismember the community and trigger or encourage development of an intertwined nexus of possibly reinforcing pathologies and destructive syndromes with the gravest impact on public health and public order, particularly for control of HIV infection. (p. 893)

The implications of this notion for communities affected by violence, extreme poverty and crime are obvious, and the principle is possibly applicable to communities in developing countries, although a database sufficient for an analysis of this type is currently lacking (Wallace, 1991). The process of breakdown he describes is a disempowering process for women (in this context increasing the incidence of drug-related prostitution) and it could be argued that disempowerment of women has been a long term historical process in the African context, indicating longer term decline and less easily identifiable processes of social breakdown. The concept of environmental disorder was also identified by Loslier (1993) in a study of the spatial variations of health indicators in Puerto Rico, he concluded that 'the most pathogenic milieux are those which are the most difficult for the subject to understand and/or control', and that *'ambiocontrol*, the conceptual control of one's setting and course of his or her life is a fundamental determinant of health' (p. 743).

The implication that the psychosocial environment, or the degree of 'ambiocontrol' as he calls it, is a major indicator of health status, reduces the importance of other, computer-friendly indicators such as socioeconomic status or access to local health units. This paves the way for a new geography of *subjective environments* in relationship to HIV/AIDS, and this humanist concept has great bearing on the understanding of HIV epidemiology. The concept of individual control over the environment re-introduces the role of agency through the capacity to perceive, respond, and indeed, *control* the health environment. High risk situations are thus geographically and socially defined zones where the capacity of the individual to effectively respond to a

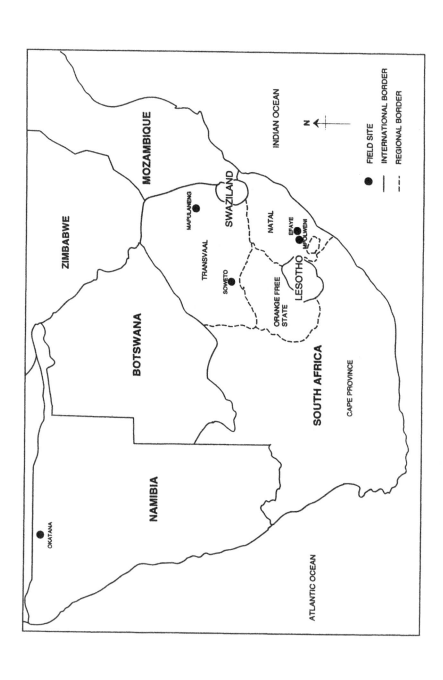

health threat is reduced. This capacity is dependent upon a host of factors, both behavioural and structural, and it is the interplay of these factors, through the actions of agency, which result in the extent of high risk behaviour in any given context. The need to identify these zones must be stressed in order to focus resources effectively – in an urban African context they may be bars, hotels, truck stops, market places, border posts, prisons, military communities, refugee camps, schools, university halls of residence and night clubs. The role of the individual though is always crucial, as HIV infection is, in a sense, a deliberate action, through the act of sexual intercourse, although transmission of the virus is usually not a deliberate reason for sexual intercourse. The aspect of choice in the decision-making process is highly complex, and in contrast to other diseases such as tuberculosis or malaria, prevention is ultimately a behavioural action.

The interaction of structures and agency, in creating the epidemiology of HIV, has geographical variation. This interaction occurs in zones of regionalisation, or in *places*. Phenomenological understanding of perception, in the creation of a sense of place, would be a variable in determining behaviour. How individuals behave changes according to their sense of place of whatever location they are in. The behaviour of a migrant labourer may be very different in a township as compared to the rural setting, in both an absolute and phenomenological sense. People's sense of rationality changes according to where they are and what they are doing. Drunk men leaving bars late at night for example will have different attitudes towards sex and risk taking than when they are sitting at their office desk during the day. Cruel examples of sexual abuse and exploitation are so often linked to alcohol that bars and the immediate surrounding areas must be one of the main points of intervention, but for some reason they are so often ignored in education campaigns in favour of less socially sensitive areas, such as hospital waiting rooms or corridors in public buildings.

Field Sites

The five field sites for the investigation are shown in Figure 2.3, and cover the geographical areas of the eastern Transvaal (now the Province of Mpumalanga), Soweto and the Natal Midlands in

Figure 2.3 *opposite* Location of the field sites

South Africa, together with the communal lands in northern Namibia (formerly known as Owamboland). The sites are geographically defined as communities, and are villages in all but one case, that of the locality of Pimville in Soweto. As the fieldwork was conducted before the April 1994 elections and the subsequent redrawing of territorial boundaries, the former homelands are referred to throughout the text. Restructuring has since rendered the homeland boundaries obsolete, along with their administrations, which survive in a modified form as regional authorities. Only one field site (consisting of the villages of Boelang and Moloro) are located within a former homeland (Lebowa). The field sites were chosen as being accessible to academic institutions – each site is linked to research institutions in some way. This fact enabled the rapid review of literature related to each site and researchers previously active in those sites – existing information sources provided valuable baseline data. Without these linkages the field work in five, rather than fewer sites within a twelve month period would have been impossible.

Moloro/Boelang, Mapulaneng, Lebowa

These two adjacent villages in the Brooklyn District of Mapulaneng, Lebowa are typical of the villages in this eastern Transvaal *lowveld* area (Figure 2.4). The 25 villages within Mapulaneng have many female headed households, as the proportion of males who are migrant labourers is relatively high. One study in the Bushbuckridge area (which incorporates the adjacent former Gazankulu region of Mhala) found that 60 per cent of males aged 30–49 were migrant labourers.[6] The average household size is around seven people, with household income at around R520 per month.[7] Over half of the household expenditure is on food. Unemployment is high, at approximately 40–50 per cent, and approximately 50–75 per cent of families depend on income received from men working in distant urban areas. The area is characterised by poverty, differential access to water (35 per cent of households are one kilometre or more away from the nearest water point), and a small amount of subsistence agriculture. Individual plots are small (average of 0.25 hectares), owing to a high population density. The foremost health care structure in the area is Tintswalo Hospital in the town of Acornhoek, seven kilometres away. At the time of the fieldwork, this hospital fell under the jurisdiction of Gazankulu authorities, but in reality the Lebowan population

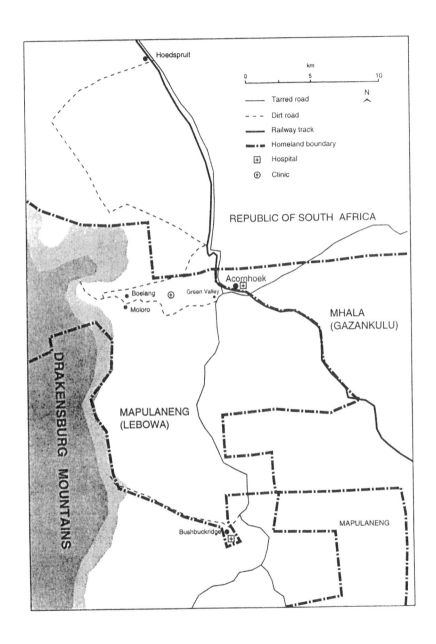

Figure 2.4 Lebowan field site (Boelang and Moloro) in context

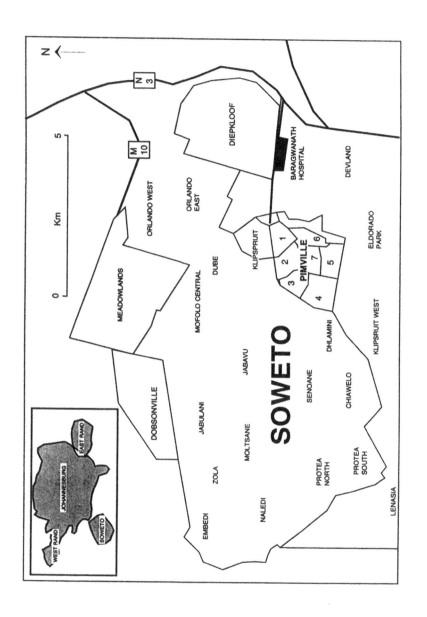

within Mapulaneng was served also, through both medical services and extension work in the form of sexual health education
and mobile clinics.

Pimville, Soweto, Transvaal
Pimville has a total of seven zones and an estimated population
of 56,000, with an average of around six people per dwelling.
Income and socioeconomic status vary across Pimville, with
Zones 2 and 3 being two of the lower class zones. Several families
often occupy one plot, with the garage and a metal shack in the
back yard often inhabited. Zone 5 is one of the more recent
additions to Pimville and has good quality housing occupied
mainly by nuclear families. Baragwanath Hospital provides the
main health care for Soweto, but Pimville also has its own clinic.
Households were randomly selected within the sample area, and
interviews were conducted with the assistance of two field-work-
ers in Pimville, Zones 2, 3 and 5. Languages used were English,
Sotho, Tswana and Zulu. The Pimville site is shown in the
context of greater Soweto in Figure 2.5.

Mpolweni Mission and Efaye, New Hanover, Natal
Two field sites were chosen from the New Hanover Magisterial
district, the communities of Mpolweni Mission, in the south-west
of the district, and Efaye Tribal Authority, in the north-east of
the district (Figure 2.6). The sites were chosen after discussion
with health care workers in the area, as these two sites have good
data bases providing socioeconomic information regarding the
communities.

In the community of Mpolweni Mission, roughly 25 kilometres north-west of Pietermaritzburg, the land is owned by
the Reformed Presbyterian Church and was formally part of
the Church of Scotland. Residents must meet strict criteria
before being allowed to live on the land. They must be Presby-
terians, be married, and have been married in a Christian
ceremony. Recently these criteria have been less strictly ad-
hered to, but the process is still stringent. Tenants pay R80
per year in rent for approximately 0.4 hectares of land. Water
costs are R60 per year per household. A programme is being
mooted to increase owner occupation in the area but this is
receiving opposition from the church. There are other religious

---

Figure 2.5 *opposite* Pimville in context

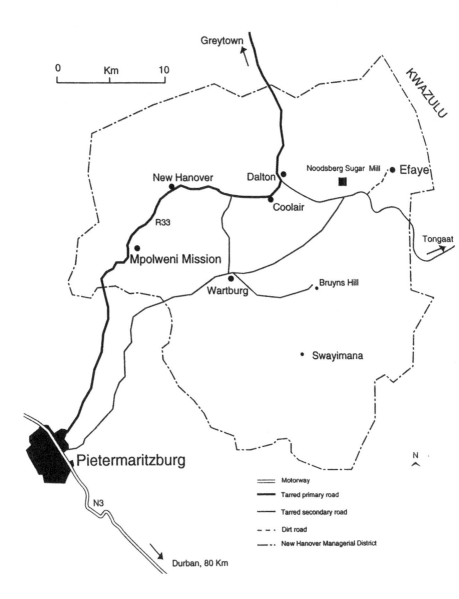

Figure 2.6 Natal field sites (Mpolweni Mission and Efaye) in context

affiliations in the area, such as Zionists, but these are frowned upon and eviction and even violence has been threatened. Traditional healers are present but their influence is limited. People use the formal health care structures available to them. A new clinic was completed in 1993 under the auspices of the Department of National Health and Population Development (DNHPD) and functions as the only formal health care structure in the area. Before this time, a mobile clinic from Pietermaritzburg was the only facility. The community as a whole has a healthy profile; there have only been two to three cases of tuberculosis in recent years. The area covers 2,200 hectares with 680 *registered* households. The population is estimated to be around 8,000. Families are most commonly extended. The community is very conservative, and no liquor is allowed to be sold on the mission, but there are known *shebeens* in the area. Mpolweni is a very closed community, and relatively unique within the New Hanover area, due to its mission status.

The second Natal field site, Efaye, is a more typical New Hanover rural settlement. The average household monthly income is around R400, and only 7 per cent of sample households earn more than R1,000 per month; the workforce is involved mainly with agricultural work on nearby sugar cane farms. The status of the land was under dispute; it was unclear whether the land was under state or Kwazulu jurisdiction. The debate is now obsolete since the 1994 election, as the land is now officially within the Kwazulu/Natal Province. The population is estimated to be around 12,500 with an average of ten family members per household. The community has a poorer health profile than Mpolweni due to the higher incidence of poverty, and access to health services is again very poor. A mobile clinic visits every two weeks and this is deemed totally inadequate for the needs of the community. The nearest permanent formal health care structure is in Mtulwa, a round trip costing R3-60, or there is a clinic in Dalton; a round trip costing R5. The community is very traditional regarding beliefs and customs, and there is a strong social support system within the community. Religious affiliations are Lutheran (80 per cent) and Zionist Christian (5 per cent).[8]

Okatana, Oshana Region, Namibia
The 'village' of Okatana is situated approximately five kilometres north of Oshakati (Figure 2.7). The settlement is very dispersed and identified only by the Roman Catholic mission hospital

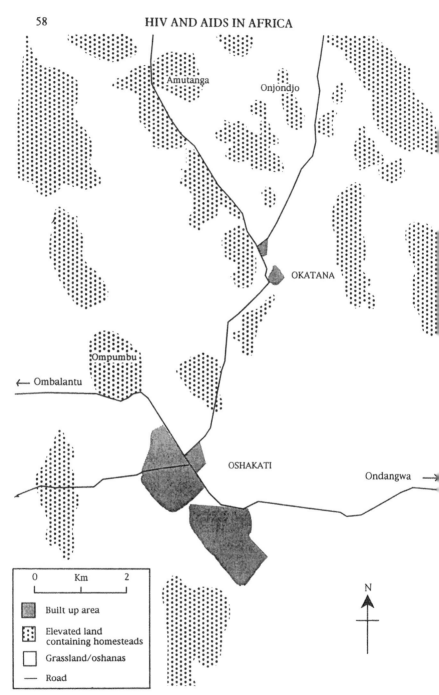

Figure 2.7 Namibian field sites (around Okatana) in context

together with a high school. Due to the flat topography of the area and abundance of surface water during the wet season, the dominant settlement type is dispersed, linked together by a series of small service centres. There is also a small collection of *cuca* and other shops close to the hospital, where formal and informal trading takes place. The people who use this small service centre live in homesteads scattered around the adjacent area. Homesteads are restricted to slightly elevated land which surrounds the small pans or *oshanas* which flood periodically. The land around the homesteads is mostly cultivated with the local variety of millet, *omahangu*, while some small scattered orchards also exist. Okatana is surrounded by smaller settlement centres such as Ompumbu to the south-west and Onjondjo to the north. The sample was divided between residents of Okatana, Onjondjo, Ompumbu and students at Amutanga Secondary School. All these locations are dormitory to Oshakati, both for services and employment, and cannot be separated functionally from this large service and military centre and now district headquarters. There are no reliable estimates of population for this area, but the sample frame in this study is somewhere in the region of 5,000 people. Data were again collected through 100 semi-structured interviews with community residents, during June and July 1993. Respondents were randomly selected within the sample area, and interviews were conducted with the assistance of a nurse from Okatana Roman Catholic Hospital. The questions were open-ended and took place in a variety of settings: at homesteads, a school, in cuca shops and at the hospital itself. A separate questionnaire study was conducted amongst school students in the Oshakati/Ondangwa nexus.

A summary of the field sites with these structural indicators is in Table 2.1 overleaf. The information comes from the 528 interviews conducted across the five sites, along with local sources which are referenced below.

Methodological Considerations

The question of knowledge is fundamental to the examination of the subject–environment interaction in relation to HIV epidemiology. Two major areas of enquiry are thus needed: an 'objective' analysis of the context of HIV spread, and the subjective environment of individuals' perceptions and behaviour, to form a construct of the nature of their interrelationship. Methodological precedents for such an examination are lacking in this respect, as Ankrah (1989) noted:

> Researching AIDS sets the social scientist, as it does the medical and biological researchers, on a largely uncharted course. As the disease has spread, it has become clearer that the factors relevant to understanding it are varied. This calls for a thorough re-examination of social science methodology. (p. 270)

Table 2.1. Economic and demographic indicators of sample communities.

Site	Population	Average household size	Sample dependency ratio[a]	Average household income (R per month)	Unemployment rate (%)
Moloro/ Boelang	6,000	7	3.5[b]	c.500	c.50[c]
Pimville	56,000	5	2.4	c.1000	c.40
Mpolweni	8,000	8[d]	3.6	c.800	c.60
Efaye	12,500	10	4.0	c.400	c.65
Okatana	5,000	10	6.7	c.500	c.50

a   Defined as the ratio of consumers to those in paid employment. Those who are unemployed are classed as dependants, even if they are seeking work. Some households have no members in the formal sector, or are completely reliant on pensions. In other households all members are economically active.
b   Estimate.
c   Health Situation Analysis, 1992, Health Services Development Unit, unpublished.
d   This figure is derived from the breakdown of the sample households. The manager of the mission estimates the figure to be 10–11.

The lack of a precedent creates problems in turning a conceptual framework into a workable methodology. Traditional methods are either quantitative or qualitative in design, possibly excluding certain variables from analysis, such as belief systems regarding disease aetiology, which requires an essentially humanistic research approach, and an overall immersion in the subjective. Disciplinary boundaries are meaningless in HIV/AIDS research, as HIV transmission, as an objective phenomenon, lies at the junction of various overlapping disciplinary systems: historical, sociological, economic, cultural, political, anthropological and virological. Providing a methodological framework for the study of such a diversity of variables, as well as their interaction, is a problem not yet resolved by epidemiologists and social scientists.

With a methodological division of the study into the interrelationship of individual and environment, different areas of knowledge are addressed which require different approaches. The research data upon which this book is based draws upon three unit scales of direct study: the individual, the household and the community. The behaviour of the individual is constrained by both household and community, and this book explores their interrelationship with reference to a response to a common threat (the HIV/AIDS epidemic) which has differential impact and its own subjective geographies. At larger scales, i.e. the region and nation, secondary sources of information are referred to (Figure 2.8).

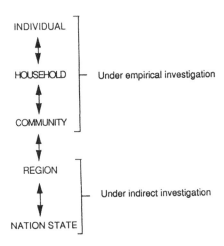

Figure 2.8. Scales of analysis

The underlying assumption is made that the overall response is partly constructed at all scales, with resultant conflicts between individuals, males and females, the 'community ethos' and policy makers.

The definition of community in this sense refers to the geographically defined group with constant internal interaction, whose individuals recognise their own membership to the community, and who have a shared life context with 'mutual accountability' (Campbell, 1990; Butchart and Seedat, 1990). Larger scale communities are examined in relation to the macro-responses to the epidemic, and a continual reference to scale, context and indeed conflict, are essential to a geographical understanding of the epidemic:

> A full rendering of the AIDS epidemic in a particular location thus places it in local, regional, and national contexts and, in some cases, the geopolitics of competing international communities. (Herdt and Lindenbaum, 1992, p. 330)

Only the micro-scale was researched in an empirical sense, but no attempt is made to differentiate between the scales of analysis in terms of importance in determination. The study attempts to evaluate the linkages between the different levels of influence, and how these linkages vary geographically. The structure–agency interaction requires the recognition of flexible *duality* and the rejection of the notion that the shape of the epidemic is either wholly structurally determined, or a result of the collective actions of agents at any given scale. To examine this duality, the intermediate levels of household and community are thus introduced as media for the interaction of agent and structure. The structures under investigation (any defined conditions of the socioeconomic environment which in some way influence HIV epidemiology) are in a sense *aspatial* as they are manifest at all scales of interaction. 'Culture' may have a set of definitions at a regional scale but become more diffuse at the community–household–individual level. Different individuals will accord differently with cultural norms through their behaviour, by either conscious resistance/conformity (purposive action) or through subconsciously motivated action which either reinforces or threatens the continued existence of that particular cultural definition. The value of Giddens' conceptualisation is thus realised when examining behaviour in relation to both its motivations and consequences.

Attempting a quantitative, survey-based study, confronts the problem of investigating sexual behaviour on a wide scale. Research of this type is valuable if done correctly, but is strewn with ethical pitfalls which have to be accounted for. Knowledge, attitude and belief are variables which are difficult to define, let alone study with any degree of accuracy. Information from the respondent regarding sexual behaviour may be highly distorted or simply not forthcoming, implying that more qualitative designs that utilise anthropological research methods, convenience samples, key actors and focus groups, may be more appropriate. Theory formation, though, requiring the testing of hypotheses, may need large quantitative surveys *supplemented* with qualitative data. But, as Standing (1992) points out, small scale, in-depth research is not 'ungeneralisable' by definition, as its wider relevance depends on the criteria of selection. In this context, defining social and cultural parameters of a case group is imperative. Previous records and key informants can provide this information, which can act as a sound base upon which to embark on questionnaire work. The aim of the precise research project may in fact determine scale and thus methodology, as Ulin observes (1992, p. 69):

> Qualitative field methods have the advantages of more open and flexible data collection techniques, as well as allowing an inductive approach to the development of a grounded theory on AIDS-specific behaviour where few hypotheses have been formulated, much less tested. On the other hand, the importance of hypothesis testing and replicability of scientific findings must not be overlooked. The best resolution to these difficult issues may be a combination of hypothesis-generating studies using a wide range of exploratory techniques, and larger surveys carefully designed to take advantage of insights from prior qualitative investigation.

The argument here is that larger quantitative work should follow in the wake of smaller qualitative studies. The findings of these smaller studies will very often provide conflicting data and a pattern only emerges when several studies are examined together. The collection of basic data can include the examination of the interaction between variables in the minds of the agents. The geographic element of the research must be maintained throughout, as Kearns and Joseph (1993, p. 716) suggested:

Clearly, the implications for design and method are profound: an engagement with the researched groups and their place (both physical and societal) is essential in the (re)construction of the relationship between people, place and health experience.

The methodology of data collection in my case conformed with the principles of Rapid Assessment Procedures (RAP) (Manderson and Aaby, 1992) which is flexible and exploratory in nature. The bulk of the information was acquired through semi-structured, open-ended, questionnaire interviews. The efficacy of the questionnaire interview as a technique to extract reliable information on sociosexual attitudes and behaviour has been questioned, because 'they ignore much of what psychoanalysis has discovered about resistance and unconscious process' (Abramson, 1992, p. 108). Abramson presses for the re-examination of insights gained from psycho-analytical tests (those which directly explore the subconscious processes of the subject) within an ethnographic framework, using a team of ethnographers to triangulate data and overcome the inherent sampling biases. My sample size was over 500 people, and considering the time constraints involved in the study, such in-depth analysis was impossible, and for research of this type the WHO claims that the structured, face to face interview is the most efficient way to obtain information about sexual behaviour (Schopper et al., 1993).

The use of a local interpreter is essential in this respect to enable access into the communities and into the lives of community residents. The sample frame was decided upon in conjunction with the interpreter who was best positioned to locate the boundaries of the 'community' area. Where the researcher's initial familiarity with the community is inadequate, consultation with a local person is necessary to draw up these perceptual boundaries, which may contradict administrative boundaries found on maps of the area. This is especially relevant in work in urban areas, where different ethnic groups often cluster together within a compound setting for example, leading to recognised but informal boundaries between sub-communities. This recognition of perceived groupings was important in the Namibian case study, where settlement morphology in the field site is dispersed and locational boundaries are ill-defined (see Figure 2.7). The interpreter on each occasion was well known to the community, and in a position to play the role of key informant. The interpreters were briefed on the design of the questionnaire and were informed on the type of information required. Points of information regarding the disease were given during our discussions between interviews. The principal problem with using a local interpreter is with the loss of anonymity between the interviewer and the interviewee. The interpreter therefore was in the ambiguous position of being neither an independent, anonymous member of the sample community, nor an outsider, due to his/her contractual arrangement with myself, the *real* 'outsider'. Responses to questions on sexual attitudes were thus given in an atmosphere tainted with some degree of personal familiarity. In the context of this research, though, this was unavoidable. Within each site a random sample of households was visited, covering as wide a geographical area as possible. The demographic structure of the sample population was decided upon in the first field site and then replicated in the following sites, to allow for inter-site comparison. A breakdown of the total sample is shown in Figure 2.9. The sample is biased towards people aged between 15 and 39, reflecting the age groups most affected by HIV and AIDS. (Figures 1.1 to 1.3).

An additional sample bias can be assumed in that the vast majority of the interviews were conducted during working hours on weekdays. As a result, a proportion of the working population is excluded from analysis, thus causing an over-representation of unemployed respondents within the sample. Migrant labourers are, therefore, also under-represented. Each interview lasted approximately 15–30 minutes, with a greater amount of time spent with respondents who were willing to discuss the issues in further detail. The refusal rate was very low, and any refusals were related to the lack of free time on the part of the respondent. The actual subject matter of the questionnaires related to local development and health issues, with specific reference to teenage pregnancy, sexually transmitted diseases (STDs) and prostitution. Any biases related to personalised information regarding sexual behaviour were avoided by using the community response rather than the personal response as the scale of enquiry. Personal whims and inclinations would still be evident, but depersonalised through the extrapolation to the community level. Focus group discussions were held in three of the five sites with adolescent school students, covering subjects related to sexual health and AIDS. The use and value of focus group discussions has been repeatedly emphasised and my motivations for the use of the group

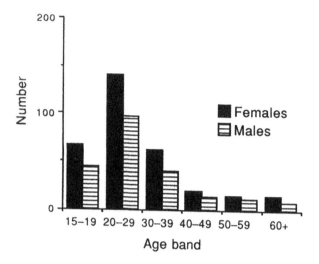

Figure 2.9. Demographic breakdown of sample respondents

discussions were twofold: as a forum for a pilot discussion in
order to define the relevant issues, and as a means of following
up, in detail, issues which became apparent during the interviews themselves, particularly in relation to transactional sex
and attitudes towards those infected with HIV (Chapters 4 and
5). Throughout the fieldwork, interviews were also conducted
with key informants, in particular medical and non-medical
personnel related to HIV/AIDS work and these are referred to
where appropriate.

During the work, the problems involved with field research
of this type were evident, but not inhibiting. The ethics involved with first world research in third world contexts is an
issue of current debate (Sidaway, 1992; Farmer, 1992 in relation to anthropology). In question are the terms of responsibility for the valid use of information acquired, and who the
research is ultimately supposed to benefit, the researcher or the
subject group. The research of sensitive issues, of which HIV/
AIDS is one (sometimes unnecessarily so), is also receiving
renewed academic attention in terms of methodological and
epistemological refinement. Affiliation with a locally recognised
body is essential, in order to attempt to overcome any suspicion of the research motive, and allay any fears of a hidden
political agenda or surreptitious association. The issues of

AIDS, politics and racial divides are discussed in detail in Chapter 3. The more immediate problem in relation to the questionnaire interviews was the issue of bias, both with the respondent and the interviewer. The most crucial issue was gender, and the reliability of the information provided, given that some of the questions related to sexual mores and attitudes. Herod (1993), outlined the areas of doubt associated with interviews and gender identities:

- How the gender of the interviewer or interviewee may shape the research process.

- How gender relations are implicated in the structure of particular research methodologies.

- How gendered assumptions can affect the way in which information generated in an interview is interpreted.

For example, men are more likely to be aggressive and engage in tall story telling, when in the company of men rather than women. In a one-to-one situation, a male respondent could engage in paternalism with a female interviewer, or in this case female interpreter, and one-upmanship with a male one. Herod noted the various stereotypes regarding linguistics; males are dominant, joke telling, blunt and lucid, while women are shy, unsure, and rarely callous. Generalising about gender relations and the influence of class and race is difficult, as the variability between respondents is so great, contributing to the overall heterogeneity regarding attitudes to both questions and the questioner. In a Knowledge, Attitude, Practice and Belief (KAPB) study in Moyo, Uganda, men did not report any overt problems in interviewing women, but it is suggested that the women under-report the number of their sexual partners when interviewed by a male (Schopper et al., 1993). In two of my five field sites (Efaye and Okatana), the interpreter used was female, but any effect this may have had on the respondents is impossible to quantify and was certainly not apparent during the interviews themselves. Questions regarding the use of condoms were answered honestly on the whole in the opinion of my translators, and our level of trust was such that blatantly false answers were often greeted with mirth and further questioning by the translator without my intervention. Another issue is that of language use. The questionnaire used in the course of the work was translated into five languages (Northern Sotho, Sotho, Zulu, Oshiwambo and Tswana) and this can create problems with word definition. Words such as 'prostitute', 'problem' and the precise definition of family members need to be investigated thoroughly before their use in a questionnaire. Experience from this research has also demonstrated the importance of community perceptions of the researcher. Even though all efforts were made to be 'independent' in the research, institutional affiliation would have inevitably led to some misconceptions regarding my motives, over and above my being a white male carrying out such work. The importance of the recognition of local conditions and constructions of knowledge is vital, and warrants much research in its own right.

A separate, but equally important, point relates to political instability and its adverse effect on field research. Cross (1990, p. 26) raised the exaggerated view of many outsiders that 'conditions in South Africa are so tense and tindery that no research operations can be carried out, due to either physical danger or social incendiarism'. Awareness of political developments and sensitivities was certainly essential at all times during the fieldwork. The political climate in South Africa has been unstable for a number of years, but recent violence has centred on the Inkatha Freedom Party (IFP)/African National Congress (ANC) conflict in Kwazulu/Natal and previous to the time of the fieldwork in the townships surrounding Johannesburg. The violence has intensified in recent years with there being over 3,000 politically motivated killings in 1993 alone (Chapter 3). The run-up to the April 1994 elections proved to be a time of great uncertainty and political tension, characterised by complete unpredictability. Two notable events during the fieldwork were the riots involving taxi drivers in Soweto during January 1993, and the time period following the assassination of South African Communist Party (SACP) leader, Chris Hani, in April 1993. Both events, characterised by localised random acts of violence, created an atmosphere of uncertainty which changed on a daily basis. Colleagues in Soweto advised me on several occasions to suspend work for the day due to outbreaks of attacks on cars driven by whites. In Natal, I was urged to suspend fieldwork for a period of several weeks following Hani's assassination due to reported attacks on vehicles in the field area. In Mpolweni in Natal, an area loyal to the ANC,[9] I was warned on a number of occasions by village leaders of the possibility of an unmotivated attack at any time, possibly not within the village, but certainly in its immediate surrounds. In Efaye, an area loyal to the IFP, the local *induna* advised me to be clear of the village by dusk. The reality of dangers during fieldwork were made evident by the highly publicised killing of an American student, Amy Biehl, in the Cape Town township of Guguletu in August 1993, supposedly by supporters of the Azanian People's Liberation Army (APLA), the military wing of the Pan Africanist Congress (PAC). This horrific killing was labelled as 'a grim parable of what happens when white liberalism meets black racism'.[10] However, at no one time did I feel directly threatened by any situation, as the dangers of my working conditions were, to a point, mitigated by affiliations with respected bodies. The sporadic nature and unpredictability of the violence at this time instilled both a nature of fatalism, combined with opportunism for research in a dynamic and stimulating, if potentially dangerous context.

3 The Political Economy of AIDS in Southern Africa: the Macro-Determinants

The examination of the HIV/AIDS epidemic at its various geographical scales, from individual through to household, community, nation and region, is imperative if a holistic picture is to be drawn. Explanations of perceptions at an individual scale are often to be found in structures of the political economy. The macro-responses to the epidemic in southern Africa: the actions of governments, health structures and the organisations which wield influence over the health of people, such as the large scale industries or unions, have been formed in a context which is generally restrictive to the planning of an adequate HIV/AIDS policy. The nature of this context is the subject of this chapter; it is important also to understand which features of this context have a direct impact on the formulation of programmes, their implementation and ultimately their success or failure.

The responses of governments, in particular, have come under close scrutiny, and in relation to South Africa the verdict of academic analysts has been one of criticism (Zwi and Bachmeyer, 1990; Christie, 1991; Hamilton, 1991; Fleming, 1992; Holmshaw, 1992; Van Niftrik, 1992; Strachan, 1992; Carswell, 1993). This needs justification, in the light of the understanding of the context in which health planning decisions were made. A host of influences on governments, from drought, economic structural adjustment programmes (ESAPs), to political upheaval and prejudice, along with some strong suggestions of enlightened self-interest, combined to de-prioritise the HIV/AIDS epidemic in both the minds and the pockets of key decision makers. At the same time, the question must also be asked whether it was at all possible to formulate an appropriate policy, given both the nature of the disease and the structural inertia of social factors such as oscillatory migration and existing health care services. In South Africa, the focus of attention in this chapter, the inadequacy of the governmental response is most starkly evident, but again what real opportunities to halt the epidemic were either apparent or achievable? As Alan Fleming, who was based at Baragwanath Hospital in Soweto for some years noted: 'Professor Ruben Sher in reviewing the present situation says that South Africa has lost the battle to prevent AIDS. I disagree: the battle was never joined' (1992, p. 428). In understanding the epidemic, the role of key organisations in influencing people's behaviour is vital, and lessons learned can be implemented at a local level in order that hospitals, local government, NGO and community based organisation (CBO) activity can have maximum impact in preventing the spread of HIV.

This chapter will explore the policy responses to the epidemic within the context in which they were formulated, and qualify the accusation of irresponsibility often placed on decision makers across the whole of the region. A balanced account must consider the restrictions placed on the ability of institutions to react in an adequate way, as well as the economic and political climate contextualising the responses.

Governmental Response

The spread of HIV/AIDS has been mostly unhindered in southern Africa, and it is reasonable to propose that governmental intervention in the region has had very little impact on the course of the epidemic. There are two possible explanations for this: first, that governments' responses were too inadequate in formulation, extent and timing to have had any impact on the spread of HIV; second, it can be argued that the complex nature of the epidemic required an institutional response beyond the means and resources of governments. An analysis of the situation in South Africa and more widely in southern Africa reveals that both of these explanations are equally applicable. Cultural relativity must also be considered when analysing responses to the epidemic. This applies both to the cultural context of HIV infection and the manifestations of the different cultural constructions of the disease:

> If an earthquake – or an epidemic like AIDS – is conceptualised as a natural disaster, an act of God, people in some cultures are less likely

to expect or demand immediate government assistance than if it is seen as a massive social or public health crisis (in other cultures, the opposite might be true). (Treichler, 1992, p. 87)

Governmental responses in the region generally took shape around 1987, when the period of denial started to be eroded by a more widespread acceptance of a growing health crisis. Under the auspices of the World Health Organization, governments allocated scant resources to newly created National AIDS Control Programmes (NACPs). These were usually creatures of the various ministries of health, some enjoying more degrees of autonomy than others.

In Namibia, organised response since independence has taken the form of the NACP initiated following independence from South Africa in April 1990. The NACP is partly funded by WHO and is nominally independent of the Ministry of Health. The South West Africa People's Organisation (SWAPO) had formulated short term programmes with the assistance of the WHO prior to formal independence. A five-year programme was proposed in 1990, and 60 donors pledged R6m (about £1.2m) for the first year. It has established regional AIDS action committees, which in 1994 did not incorporate NGOs. Since July 1991, the NACP has promoted the annual National Safe Sex Promotion Week and commissioned a national awareness survey (NISER, 1991).

In Botswana, governmental response was relatively rapid, with blood screening taking full effect in 1986. In 1987, the government, in conjunction with the WHO, implemented a one year short term plan which was followed two years later by a five year medium term plan. The country now has its second medium-term plan (MTP2) – another five year programme. This took the form of education programmes involving posters by roadsides, on which it spent US$170,000 per year.[1] A comprehensive STD control programme has been strengthened, again with WHO funds. A promising development in Botswana, which is also occurring in Zimbabwe, Zambia and Swaziland, and is certainly encouraged in South Africa, is the integration of traditional healers into the formal health education system. Seminars attended by both traditional healers and regional health team workers provide a forum for interaction and mutual education. Diseases tackled have been STDs, tuberculosis and infant diarrhoea. These meetings have been running successfully since 1979 in Botswana (Haran, 1991). Although Botswana's national health system is relatively well developed, labour shortages in some areas have impeded progress, but overall public awareness has grown. Lessons are still being learned; for example a trial of 15 vending machines selling condoms in Gaborone has been declared a failure due to mechanical faults.[2]

Government response has been fairly similar in Zimbabwe; a medium term plan initiated in 1988 with a budget of US$13m, funded primarily by the now defunct Global Programme on AIDS (GPA) in Geneva. This plan was formulated despite much initial reluctance to admit the presence of the disease. The Government of Zambia formally recognised the problem in 1987 but has been hampered by financial restrictions throughout. Governmental commitment to tackling the disease in Zambia is still patchy. Katele Kalumba, the Minister of Health, claimed he was fighting a 'lone battle' within the government in mobilising action and resources from government coffers as recently as 1995.[3] In Mozambique, a NACP has been nominally in place since 1988, but the civil war has prevented any wide scale opportunities for intervention. Peaceful conditions following the elections in 1994 hopefully herald a new period of active intervention.

Governmental Response in South Africa

Of all the countries in the southern African region, the response of South Africa to the AIDS epidemic has been the one most characterised by denial, ministerial wrangling, the misallocation of resources, and has been muted throughout by those forces either resisting or pushing for political transformation. Nowhere have the polemics of the AIDS debate, fuelled by media hysteria, taken on such political colourings, and nowhere have the interests surrounding a disease been so related to existing patterns of power between and within social groups. When the first deaths from AIDS in South Africa occurred in 1985, it was apparent that action of some form had to be taken. What was not anticipated by NGOs was a systematic neglect of the HIV/AIDS epidemic and refusal to take responsible action for those at risk from infection; a neglect which was first reacted to by the gay community. The meagre R1m (about £200,000) spent in 1985 was squandered on an education campaign depicting coffins in graves; 'the general perception seemed to be that the scene portrayed a victim of political violence' (Van Niftrik, 1992, p. 1).

This was followed, in a later campaign, by skeletons as bed partners of amorous couples, leaving the population even more confused than before. Rumours of political plots were rife. After all, the South African administration had had little credibility with the majority of the people regarding matters sexual, ever since the disastrous 'baby for Botha' campaign in 1967, in which white families were requested to have one more baby than originally planned in an effort to dispel Malthusian fears in government ranks. Conversely, evidence from Namibia indicates that there was widespread use of DepoProvera injections by health staff on black women, often without their knowledge or consent, as a 'population control' policy (Lindsay, 1989).

The politicising of the AIDS epidemic did not take long. The Conservative Party blatantly ignored the known facts about the disease to scaremonger the white population. Right wing groups claimed that AIDS was synonymous with returning ANC cadres trained in countries further north, particularly Zambia (Zwi and Bachmeyer, 1990). Meanwhile the government 'handled' the situation in 1987 by proclaiming AIDS a communicable disease, thus condoning the official quarantining of those even suspected to be HIV-positive. This was never actually carried out but the legislation provided for it. The maintenance of the status quo was the government's first priority; ignoring the epidemic was the policy to that effect. The ANC initially skirted the issue, only having to face up to the problem when calls for the HIV testing of returning ANC exiles, especially Umkhonto weSizwe (MK) guerrillas formerly resident in Angola, were headline news. The ANC objected to any testing of the estimated 40,000 returnees from Zambia, Uganda, Angola and Tanzania, all areas of high HIV prevalence. The ANC later explained their initial laxness on any sort of policy as being due to the 'relative unclarity about the disease' and because AIDS was related to the sexuality of people and was thus a taboo subject for political parties to address (Crewe, 1992). Only here did the ANC and the government have something to agree on.

By 1990, the ANC had started to realise that AIDS was going to be a feature of South Africa for the foreseeable future, and doomsday forecasting from some observers galvanised action in the form of the Maputo Conference, which heralded the start of any serious prevention efforts within South Africa (Stein and Zwi, 1990). Any signs of change on government policy were dismissed in 1991 when the Department of National Health and

Population Development (DNHPD) proclaimed that the promotion of condoms would encourage promiscuity (this is an objection which is often raised, but all evidence points to the opposite effect). When, in 1992, the government wasted more money on a school AIDS-education campaign which it then withdrew without reason, the credibility of the DNHPD reached its nadir and the department lost two of its most prominent figures. Wilson Carswell left for England in disgust while Amanda Holmshaw, its director, was transferred and resigned soon afterwards. AIDS education was deemed to be the domain of the ten AIDS Training, Information and Counselling Centres (ATICCs) which were established at this time. Not one of them was located in a black area, and AIDS education for the majority of the people meant the notorious 'yellow hand campaign' which further discredited any efforts on the part of the government. The large illustration of a yellow hand outline, accepted because of its supposed cultural neutrality, was actually associated with the rubber washing gloves of the 'madams', and was regarded with contempt from the outset by black South Africans. Posters produced were culturally illiterate, featuring white characters with the faces coloured in, and only rarely in the appropriate language. Pamphlets educating about AIDS prevention were printed in English and Afrikaans only, while taxis in Soweto, driven by men 'trained in AIDS prevention' carried government stickers with the message 'You cannot get AIDS from swimming pools'. Commentators continually pointed to the covert, but not so hidden agendas within education efforts:

> The national media campaign directed at black audiences is different from that designed for white audiences. Programmes designed for black audiences emphasise the debilitation and death arising from AIDS in a drastic way. For whites in contrast, the campaign is 'soft', with an emphasis on long-term love that should override short sighted unsafe sexual practices.[4]

Until 1993, sex education incorporating AIDS was put in a 'life skills context'. Unfortunately, this use of metaphor and abstract rhetoric in education programmes, rather than clear, lucid language, rendered the programmes useless, especially when the target audience comprised schoolchildren. In the Cape area, efforts by the Medical Research Council at AIDS education in schools through its 'Roxy' magazine were well received by the children but rejected by many teachers, claiming it to be too explicit, despite its adherence to WHO guidelines (Everett, 1992). Meanwhile, overt AIDS education, finally in place in schools in the Transvaal in 1993, was so moralistic in tone as to be meaningless to many students. The reputation of the Department of Health was thus also under question, as the ingrained conservatism, causing the department to be 'rooted in the past' has prevented any successful initiatives from being taken, while sex education remains firmly taboo. Condom advertising had been limited throughout, and only from 1992 was minimal promotion permitted on late night television. In the mid 1990s drives in the condom market are realising increased sales but still well below what would be expected. Australia's condom market is four times the size of South Africa's, despite comparable population sizes.[5] Controversy over AIDS education continued into the new administration. In early 1996 R14m was spent by the government on the development of an AIDS education play *Sarafina II*. This figure represents one fifth of the annual AIDS budget and the total cost of the entire annual provincial AIDS allocation.[6] The issue was not so much the content or quality of the play, but the enormous fees and eventual high cost of the producers and actors. Media attention focused on this purportedly unjustified enormous expenditure.

Government spending on AIDS has been arguably minimal, with the budget hardly exceeding that of its neighbouring countries: 1990–91, R5.4m; 1991–92, R15.3m; 1992–93, R20.9m; 1993–94, R21.1m. Zambia's AIDS budget, for example, was US$5m for 1991, three times that of South Africa. Even Mozambique, racked by civil war, was reputedly spending twice as much on AIDS education as South Africa (Hamilton, 1991, p. 6). Considering South Africa's considerable GDP per capita relative to other countries in southern Africa, the disparity in spending is even more marked. South Africa budgeted for a spending of 18 US cents per capita on the AIDS control programme (1993–94) compared to 31 US cents in Namibia (1993), 41 in Tanzania (1991), 48 in Botswana (mean per annum 1988–92), 60 in Zambia (1991) and 93 in Zimbabwe (1992–93) (Schneider and McIntyre, 1994). In 1993, the AIDS Centre of the South African Institute for Medical Research in Johannesburg was forced to close due to lack of funding, and financial restrictions on the extent of voluntary HIV testing has been carried over into the new administration.[7] As Wilson Carswell, a now outspoken critic on government policy noted; 'AIDS prevention no longer exists, except as a window dressing, and health department officials now claim that

AIDS is "the responsibility of individuals", i.e. the government no longer sees itself as having any responsibilities in this area' (1993, p. 132).

In 1992, the government finally enlisted the help of the ANC, the major unions and various non-governmental organisations to form the National AIDS Convention of South Africa (NACOSA), to coordinate and direct policy on AIDS. The pomp and ceremony of the gatherings (bolstered by a convincing speech given by Nelson Mandela) was overshadowed once again by the political in-fighting of the various actors, and the final session of the two day meeting descended into a political slanging match concerning the representativeness of the NACOSA steering committee. The government's Minister of Health, Dr Rina Venter, was notable by her absence throughout. By its second meeting in 1993, little progress had been made and NACOSA was still deemed to be a talking shop by observers. Its survival into the new majority-rule era was guaranteed in the short term at least by the drafting of the National AIDS Plan for South Africa 1994–1995 (NACOSA, 1994).

The Response of Non-Governmental Organisations (NGOs)

The role of NGOs as institutions seeking to effect change, both behavioural and structural, is crucial in the response to HIV/ AIDS. In May 1990, the Southern African Network of AIDS Service Organisations (SANASO) was formed in Harare, with the aim of integrating the work of previously disparate working groups.[8] Indeed, the growth of NGO activity has to be seen as the development of an information network, often viewed with suspicion by governments, who fear usurpation in some sectors. Their role in the effort to halt the spread of AIDS and mitigate its effects will prove vital as government response remains mixed and in general under-funded. Since 1991, Namibia has had the Namibian Network AIDS Service Organisation (NAN-ASO) which coordinates NGO activities and liaises with NACP. Similar organisations have been formed in Zambia (the Zambia National AIDS Network) and Malawi. There were 53 NGO 'implementing organisations' and 26 'support groups' working on AIDS in Zimbabwe in 1995, according to ZAN/ SAFAIDS, but the lack of cohesion between them has meant that education campaigns have been problematic. Feuding and the lack of consistency on issues such as condoms and resource use unfortunately prevent NGOs presenting a united forum in the battle against AIDS. Efforts in Tanzania have also been hampered by a lack of communication and organisation. As in Botswana, traditional healers are being utilised to complement the formal health education system in Zimbabwe, and there have been a number of large conferences with the aim of exchanging and disseminating information. Oxfam, in particular, has been supporting the Zimbabwean National Association of Traditional Healers (ZINATHA), which surveys beliefs and curative practices, implementing findings into subsequent education programmes.

Non-Governmental Response in South Africa

In South Africa, there has been much positive work done by the NGO sector, notably Gary Friedman's 'Puppets against AIDS', the activism of the AIDS Consortium and the work of the Progressive Primary Health Care Network (PPHCN), to name but a few. Unfortunately these programmes, invaluable as they are, have had very little impact on the epidemic to date. Indeed, some initiatives are fraught with problems, some political, some financial. For example, when the 'Puppets against AIDS' staged a performance at the main campus of the University of the Witwatersrand in Johannesburg in July 1992, the audience was almost exclusively white, despite the college having roughly even numbers of black and white students.[9] Another case in point is the Society for AIDS Families and Orphans (SAFO) in Soweto. Funding was received from the British Council for a vehicle, while assistance from the DNHPD was very late in coming, and indeed had been refused for some years. The United States Agency for International Development (USAID), which spent over US$74m in 1991 (Mann et al., 1992, p. 802) also refused funding for SAFO, covertly on the grounds that the coordinator of the project at the time was white, and therefore 'politically incorrect'.[10] The reputation of USAID in Africa in terms of its AIDS prevention work is tainted with accusations by analysts of hidden political agendas and assumed strong connections with American foreign policy, along with such contentious issues as targeting of funds away from AIDS and TB treatment, and the reluctance to fund blood transfusion services, both of which are vital in HIV/AIDS prevention (Turshen, 1992). In South Africa,

USAID's funding targets AIDSCOM,[11] which has had extremely mixed success, both in terms of its image and with the execution of policy. At a seminar involving AIDS education with traditional healers in Botha's Hill, Natal, jointly organised by AIDSCOM and the PPHCN, undercurrents of (black) racism, along with the accusation that the whites present (myself included) were being culturally ignorant and disrespectful, resulted in the traditional healers present at the seminar writing a letter of protest to the AIDSCOM representative who was seen as attempting to usurp the meeting for her own ends. Conflict between NGOS is nothing new of course but the scramble for funds with the emergence of the epidemic has led to some intense rivalries and disputes, over and above the usual unavoidable clashes of personality. These conflicts impede progress and draw attention away from the real tasks at hand. Donors are becoming increasingly sensitive to these disputes in the South African and southern African context, and hidden agendas do not remain hidden for very long.

As well as the many NGOs, academic institutions have been vocal in response to the inadequate governmental initiatives, but little has been done in terms of the development of possible intervention strategies, and research has been mainly oriented towards AIDS-impact alleviation rather than prevention, 'only a small fraction of research conducted so far has had any practical policy implication' (Broomberg, 1993, p. 35). Much of this work has been commissioned by large actuarial companies such as Metropolitan Life and Old Mutual, with a research brief which is understandably limited in scope. Similarly in Zambia several large studies were commissioned by international donors such as NORAD, SIDA and USAID, but the emphasis again was on the impact of the epidemic. These studies were no doubt valuable, but a dearth of knowledge still exists regarding prevention mechanisms and links with development processes.

Important role players throughout the emergence of the epidemic in South Africa have been the trade unions, notably the National Union of Mineworkers (NUM) and the Transport and General Workers' Union (TGWU). Pressure from unions, through the Congress of South African Trade Unions (COSATU), which held its first conference on AIDS in July 1991, has led to the drawing up of charters regarding the health rights of workers in relation to work place policies on HIV/AIDS, such as HIV testing without consent and the banning of the dismissal of a seropositive (but otherwise healthy) worker.

Today, the NUM continues to be very active in AIDS education, and is continually representing the rights of its seropositive members. A similar role is taken by the AIDS Consortium, a Johannesburg-based NGO forum, in relation to the
rights of seropositive patients, people with AIDS and a general
work place policy on AIDS. The Chamber of Mines had rejected the idea of negotiating a work place policy on AIDS
until 1992,[12] but now are becoming more active in the AIDS
field (Heywood, 1996), and are represented on the steering
committee of the NACOSA, having done a considerable about-
turn on the issue of HIV/AIDS since 1985.

As a result of institutional hesitance and inconsistency, large
scale efforts at AIDS prevention have had little effect outside of
the urban areas. Respondents in the sample Soweto community
claimed AIDS to be the biggest local health problem, while in
the two sample communities in Natal, where HIV prevalence
rates are possibly much higher, community health priorities were
perceived to be influenza, gastro-enteritis, hypertension and
tuberculosis (Chapter 6).

The Non-Prioritisation of HIV/AIDS

The spread of HIV/AIDS depends on people being at risk of
infection. Infection rates are highest in high risk situations,
re-defined here as socially and geographically defined zones
where the *capacity of the individual to respond effectively to a
health threat is reduced* (Chapter 2). Government responses, however inadequate, do not account for the rapid spread of HIV in
the region, and criticisms of (the lack of) government actions
are actually stressing the apparent neglect of assumed responsibility, rather than claiming that the epidemic is widespread
as a *direct result* of the lack of government intervention. What
should be stressed is that the conditions which create high risk
situations are institutionalised, in the form of, amongst other
things, migrant labour flows, economic relations and apartheid
structures in the case of South Africa. In addition, during this
period of HIV spread, structural issues became immediate,
overriding concerns in themselves: conflict, economic crisis
and drought. The combined effect of these macro-processes is
that the threat of HIV infection, although now universally
recognised within the region, is *not prioritised* in that concerns
which are (possibly) temporally and psychologically more

immediate become dominant, and to a large extent determine subsequent behaviour, including sexual behaviour.

Conflict and political instability
The southern African region has been racked by conflict over the past few decades, a conflict which has been termed the 'Thirty Years War for southern African independence' by the historian John Saul (Saul, 1994). Civil wars in Mozambique and Angola have prevented any meaningful prevention campaigns from getting off the ground. In Mozambique, the civil war claimed the lives of more than an estimated one million people, with more than three million internally displaced and one and a half million others fleeing the country. The situation remains (in mid 1996) extremely unstable in Angola, despite ceasefires and endless rounds of negotiations between the ruling MPLA and rebel UNITA forces. In Namibia, prevention efforts were delayed until after independence in 1990, following a long and protracted independence struggle. The whole idea of health promotion and education during a war situation is perceived to be absurd by those directly fighting in the war, the governments or factions involved in the war, and the ordinary civilians encountering violence, or the potential for violence, on a daily basis. Within Uganda, evidence suggests that the pattern of HIV infection in the early 1980s was directly related to the movement of army personnel, the centres of recruitment (to which soldiers returned periodically) and centres of contact between prostitutes and soldiers. A similar correlation has been noted for the movement of HIV and soldiers in Tanzania (Conner and Kingman, 1989). The AIDS situation will no doubt reach crisis proportions in Rwanda as a result of the civil war in 1994; before the fighting even started, antenatal clinic infection rates in Kigali were in the region of 30–35 per cent (Ntawuruhunga *et al.*, 1993). In a conflict situation human rights abuses through rape, for example, are commonplace and the psychological implications for HIV spread are considerable. Rape was reportedly a widespread occurrence involving South African Defence Force (SADF) soldiers in Owamboland in northern Namibia during occupation in the mid to late 1980s. Baldo and Cabral (1990, p. 37) identified the psychological processes operating in a low-intensity war situation, which have been widespread across southern Africa:

• Loss of the ability to think lucidly

- Loss of the ability to communicate truthfully

- Lack of sensitivity to the suffering of others

- Loss of hope amounting to dehumanisation

- Increased selective inattention

- Evasive scepticism

- Desire for revenge

Roderick Wallace's study (1993) of the social epidemiology of HIV in Harlem, New York, described the forces which lead to social disintegration within communities. This concept is applicable to low-intensity warfare situations, which strain the social networks to the point where 'normal' behaviour is suspended – what he calls a 'phase change'

```
SOCIOGEOGRAPHIC
NETWORK              <——> BEHAVIOURAL PATHOLOGY
FRAGMENTATION
```

Where violence is less in evidence but still pervades social life, such as in South Africa, with over 3,000 *political* deaths in 1993 and over 14,000 between 1990–94,[13] (the total number of murders has averaged over 20,000 per year since 1990[14]), and the politically turbulent Malawi, people's perceptions are altered, encouraging fatalism to become the most rational way of conducting daily life. Short term priorities relating to personal safety and the welfare of relatives overwhelm positive moves toward change regarding sexual behaviour. The result is a change in the localised psychosocial set of values. Why worry about the coming years when the coming weeks and months are so unpredictable? The theme is one of fatalism and the feeling of the loss of *ambiocontrol* (defined as 'the conceptual control of one's setting and course of an individual's life'; Chapter 2). The long term nature of the progression of HIV infection to full blown AIDS and death is subordinated in the rationale due to the immediacy of other life threatening environmental factors. A case in point is the series of 22 murders in 1993–94 of young boys in Mitchell's Plain, a coloured township on the outskirts of Cape Town, which only aroused short term interest in the local community of 50,000 people. A local minister commented:

Some people remain concerned at an individual level but as a community you'd think the issue had been forgotten. People get inured to horror here. They live with it every day. We have one of the highest murder rates in the world. Such is the poverty of the parents, the stresses on them, that too little time is left for them to attend to their children's needs. They're just left to go wandering around the streets alone. There's little opportunity for normal family life.[15]

A similar situation is evident in the Natal region where years of political instability and civil war have had the effect of de-prioritising the epidemic. Commentators have attempted to link the violence directly with sexual activity:

Sexual mores have disintegrated, and in their place a youth culture of sexual promiscuity bound up with anti-apartheid struggle places young women in a situation where to refuse sexual activity means being unpatriotic. (Hambridge, 1990, p. 2)

The same can be said for many of the Rand townships, where politically motivated civil disorder prevented any long term psychosocial perspectives from pervading the psyche of the population. Quoting Sizakele Nkosi of the ANC:

Our male comrades see violence against women as a minor issue, and whenever we bring it up we are accused of being radical feminists. (Armstrong, 1993, p. 8)

Political change was the only long term psychological structure apparent in the pre-election era, and even then the struggle to overthrow apartheid occurred in a temporal sequence of violent episodes, which acted as landmarks in the minds of people. The 'Struggle' was thus broken down sequentially, preventing the long term perspective, which HIV/AIDS represents, from dominating more immediate problems, be they related to violence or simply the conditions of daily living. The Centre for Peace Action at Wits estimated that Johannesburg had become the most violent city in the world, with an average of 52 people being killed daily, with an instance of rape every 83 seconds. Township violence was mainly centred on mine-hostels housing Zulu workers. Young men (typically Zulu and Xhosa) embroiled in, and perpetuating this conflict, would have had little regard for long term health risks such as HIV/AIDS, as political and tribal affiliation required *immediate* psychological commitment, despite the associated high risk of fatality. Violence in these areas has continued since the elections of May 1994, such as the murder of eleven people in Thokosa in July 1994, victims of the 'Taxi wars', which have had the effect of traumatising many children and severely impacting on their schooling performance.[16] In Kwazulu/Natal alone there have been over 1,000 politically motivated murders in the twelve months following the election.[17]

Wars also destroy economies and health care infrastructures which take years of reconstruction following the termination of the violence, and efforts at AIDS prevention understandably are considered to be low priorities. A systematic prevention programme will be absent in Angola for the foreseeable future, and even now in Mozambique, blood is not universally screened for HIV due to the lack of facilities. In South Africa, the level of priority accorded to HIV/AIDS is of crucial importance during reconstruction, and the new government, despite such commitments as housing, jobs, water, electricity and education, must carefully balance HIV/AIDS as a resource issue with more immediate, tangible concerns (Chapter 6).

Economic Restructuring
Governments not faced by war, such as those of Zimbabwe, Tanzania and Zambia, have had economic pressures which have subsumed all others. Since the early 1980s, economic structural adjustment policies (ESAPs) imposed by the International Monetary Fund (IMF) and the World Bank have dominated economic concerns. World Bank commentators claim health budgets have not been adversely affected by this restructuring (Elmendorf and Roseberry, 1993). This point is disputed, not least because user fees, such as the three dollar treatment charge introduced in Zimbabwe, have defrayed some of the costs to the consumer.[18] In Zambia decline in attendance at clinics for routine care has been dramatic, and this has been directly linked with the introduction of user fees through a nationwide 'cost-sharing' initiative (Kahenya and Lake, 1995). Health sector budgets, however, are one factor amongst many others, and may actually have little to do with HIV spread in some contexts, when economic livelihoods and the lack of employment opportunities are more important determinants:

> Economic recession and SAPs further aggravate the transmission, spread and control of HIV infection in Africa in two major ways:

directly by increasing the population at risk through increased urban migration, poverty, women's powerless and prostitution, and indirectly through a decrease in health care provision. (Sanders and Abdulrahman, 1991, p. 161)

The attention of people is focused upon food subsidies and other forms of public spending. Again, time horizons are shortened as the threat of food shortage becomes an overwhelming concern. The Lusaka food riots in 1990 and those in Harare in 1992 testify to people's reaction to the restructuring in relation to the removal of food subsidies, and the adverse nature of the impact on public welfare.

One of the outcomes of restructuring policy is the encouragement of the development of tourism. The emergence of HIV/AIDS in the mid 1980s threatened to destroy potentially lucrative tourist markets. In 1987, a Zambian newspaper admitted that it was government policy to restrict reporting of AIDS in the country (Sabatier, 1988). Tourism in Zambia hit an all time low in 1986, due in part, or so the government believed, to negative publicity surrounding the growing number of AIDS cases. Tourism was expected to overcome the financial losses incurred in the copper industry, and AIDS was viewed as an aggravating nuisance for public relations with foreign tourist markets. Not until Kaunda's announcements on AIDS in 1987, following the loss of his son to the disease, did the government make any concerted efforts at wide scale prevention. In Zimbabwe, the word 'AIDS' was forbidden on death certificates until 1989, and the Zimbabwean press has baffled observers with its anecdotal reports of AIDS in the United States and Europe, while virtually ignoring the serious AIDS situation on its very doorstep. Timothy Stamps, as the Health Minister, has made great progress in introducing a 'rational' approach to prevention and the role of the media, calling for a ban in 1994 on the reporting in the press of traditional healers claiming to have found a cure. Just such a claim caused havoc in Malawi in early 1995 where huge traffic queues and thousands of people congested the area around the home of a traditional herbalist. In Zambia, the press has devoted much space to AIDS but has failed to lead public debate on the matter. Unlike in Zimbabwe, the media have focused on local stories in relation to AIDS and have shown widespread acceptance of the disease, although the potential role in education is still yet to be fulfilled (Kasoma, 1994). In Namibia, the development of the tourist industry, particularly relating to game reserves and the opening up of the environmentally sensitive Skeleton Coast, is crucial to the development of the economy, itself in need of foreign aid following a financially crippling independence struggle with South Africa. Levels of sensitivity regarding statistics of AIDS in the country are noticeably high, and admissions that a losing battle is being fought are to be found in the Namibian press rather than in government reports. Even in 1993, AIDS was still a taboo word, and the number of personalities and leading public figures succumbing to a 'long and cruel illness' continues to grow. The reluctance of leading figures with AIDS to go public with the disease means that icons of the northern hemisphere such as Magic Johnson and Freddie Mercury still represent AIDS in the consciousness of the South African public.[19] This is a major obstacle to destigmatising the disease, and the nature of the public reaction to the inevitable deaths of ANC figureheads from AIDS in the coming years could be crucial.

The impact of the drought, 1992–93

As well as economic pressures, adversity has taken the form of the most severe drought seen by southern Africa this century. The drought of 1992–93 forced a rapid reconceptualisation of health and development priorities across the region; the threat of famine was more important than anything else. A massive food distribution programme was implemented using vast amounts of resources. Many lives were saved but many were lost also, along with thousands of head of cattle and livestock. In Lebowa, for example, an estimated 62,000 head of cattle were lost between April and October 1992.[20] Bulawayo and Harare, amongst other major towns, were so short of water that plans were drawn up to blockade the towns against huge inflows of migrants from the parched rural areas. In Kwazulu/Natal, water stocks were 30 per cent of the usual level at the end of the summer period in 1993,[21] and at one point the main water reservoir at Louis Trichardt in the northern Transvaal was only 4 per cent full.[22] The impact of drought on food productivity and livelihoods is documented elsewhere, suffice it to say here that food security was severely (and continues to be) threatened across many parts of southern Africa. Unemployment caused by the drought was estimated at 69,000 in South Africa alone, and vegetable prices rose by 31.5 per cent during the drought period, as food production fell to 15–30 per cent of the normal output.[23] The economic impact of the drought was felt at all scales; between April and July 1992, a total of

R1.5bn (about £300m) was spent by the South African government on drought relief, mostly through subsidies on the interest on farmers' debts.[24] The final figure was nearer R4bn (£800m).

At an economic level at least, these processes of climatic devastation and macro-restructuring can be conceptualised as marginalising processes, which can reinforce the establishment of high risk situations. Immediate economic necessity becomes the overriding factor in an individual's life, and the prospect of contracting a little understood disease becomes further de-prioritised (Figure 3.1).

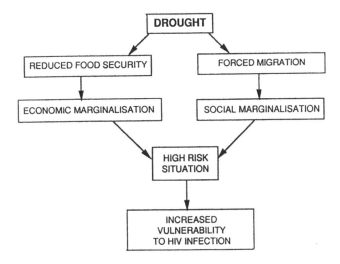

Figure 3.1. Drought and high risk situations

The proportion of the population living exclusively from subsistence agriculture in South Africa is quite low; for example, around 8 per cent in former Gazankulu (Cadman, 1987). Other sources of monetary income into the rural household budget have been affected by the drought. White farmers refused to pay wages in some areas so remittances declined, while the combined affect of sanctions and the recession have had a deleterious affect on income from industrial workers in the mines or in manufacturing. In the eastern Transvaal, this situation was exacerbated by the influx of 20,000 refugees from drought and conflict stricken Mozambique, who inevitably formed new squatter settlements or added to existing ones. Reports suggested that a cross-border slave trade was developing, as refugees were conned into prostitution and servitude in South Africa.[25] These unfortunates still claimed that even these conditions were better than those in Mozambique, where soldiers had created their own form of slave-prostitution. The implications for HIV spread under these circumstance is ominous, but AIDS is a non-issue when shelter, water and food are priorities.

In Zimbabwe, the effects of the drought were exacerbated by a change of food policy by the government. Usually, a one year supply of food is stockpiled, but under pressure from the IMF, President Mugabe gave the go-ahead for the export of this stockpile despite warnings from the maize industry that future shortages were likely. As a consequence, food rioting in Harare and Bulawayo was commonplace following the introduction of maize rationing. Crime and social violence increased, fuelled by the food shortage, which was seen as a direct consequence of the ESAP and President Mugabe's decision. Political instability, as in neighbouring Malawi, looked ever likely, and Malawi itself must now stabilise following the elections of May 1994. Mozambican refugees were being seen as competition for food handouts, and the traditional tolerance associated with rural Malawi was strained, and commentators rightly predicted increasing political turmoil, which resulted with the announcement of impending democratisation. The drought may well have been the political death knell for Dr Banda. When the rains finally did come, sanitation systems were so blocked that cholera was suddenly the primary health concern, especially in Zimbabwe and Zambia, and the threat of a major epidemic stirred panic in the health ministries of the region, even as far south as Pretoria. The result of heavy rains on parched ground and clogged sanitation systems was the worst cholera epidemic in Zimbabwe's history.[26]

As conditions deteriorated in rural areas of South Africa, especially in the northern and eastern Transvaal, thousands of people migrated in search of food, and this led to the increase in size of squatter camps around Johannesburg, Port Elizabeth and Durban,[27] and the drought has been a major factor in increasing urbanisation rates. Water rationing in Venda, for example, left some people with only a litre of water per day.[28] The twin forces of economic and social marginalisation which accompany migration renders migrants extremely vulnerable to HIV infection. Without doubt feelings of fatalism are higher amongst migrants, who would form a group at risk, with lower than average rates of condom use for example, due to unavailability, costs, and the perceived low priority of protected sex when faced with immediate and dire economic problems.

The Context of HIV/AIDS

The migrant labour system

The migrant labour system is a relic of the colonial era in southern Africa, which created a large scale demographic imbalance within both urban and rural areas. Women, entrenched in patrilineal social structures, have had a minimal role in the urban setting where they are considerably outnumbered by men, and within the job market they have often been relegated to beer selling and/or commercial sex work. The debate over the real influence of institutionalised, as well as 'voluntary' migration in southern Africa and South Africa in particular, on the social epidemiology of HIV/AIDS is apparently polarised, although the detrimental connection with general health status has received some attention (Zwi and Bachmeyer, 1990; West, 1990). With regard to HIV/AIDS, Moodie (1988), IJsselmuiden et al. (1990), Head (1992), as well as the Chamber of Mines itself (Russell, 1991), contend that the influence of the migrant labour system has in fact been exaggerated unduly. However, Jochelson et al. (1991) and – more implicitly – Abdool Karim et al. (1992), conclude that migrant labour is an important facilitator in the epidemic. Its importance, in terms of the epidemiology of HIV/AIDS, is that the virus is purported to spread from core groups (migrants and prostitutes) to the 'background' population (wives, girlfriends and rural sexual networks). The nature and extent of this mixing are not clear cut, hence the opaqueness of the debate, which still lacks any large scale informed inquiry. Studies in Zimbabwe have given contradictory results as to the direct influence of migrancy, which is applicable to between one third and one half of families. A study by Mary Bassett et al. (1993), amongst over 1,000 factory workers in Harare, showed that HIV prevalence did not differ according to household arrangements (the extent of absenteeism), despite the migrant workers engaging in higher risk behaviour. A possible explanation was that saturation level of infection had already been reached among the workforce (around 20 per cent), but this figure is relatively low, indicating that some reporter bias was at work within the sample responses, i.e. some men lied about their sexual behaviour. Indeed, the Medical Research Council in South Africa proposed a study examining the factor of migrancy on HIV/AIDS epidemiology in the Kwazulu/Natal region, then rejected it due to difficulties relating to methodology and data validation.[29] Nevertheless, Nelson Mandela drew attention to the issue in a speech to the NACOSA conference in 1992:

> Do we really have justification for perpetuating such practices as the migrant labour system and single sex hostels, which not only destroy family life, but certainly limit our capacity to establish stable, self reliant communities that form the core of a dynamic society able to cope with this and other problems? (NACOSA, 1992, p. 11)

In 1992 the Chamber of Mines employed approximately 750,000 people, the majority being male migrant workers, 98 per cent of whom lived in single sex hostels away from their families. Roughly 40 per cent of the workforce were migrant labourers from outside South Africa.[30] In a 1986 sero-survey of 30,000 black migrant mine workers conducted by the Chamber of Mines, 3.8 per cent of miners from Malawi were seropositive along with 0.3 per cent of those from Botswana. By April 1988, over 2,500 workers had been diagnosed HIV-positive (Sabatier, 1988) and the proportion of migrants from Malawi who were positive had risen from 4 per cent to 10 per cent in less than 18 months.[31] The Malawian government now does not allow migrants to work in the mines in South Africa, due to 'lack of labour at home'. The real reason is more likely to be political tension created by discrimination against Malawian migrants in South Africa.

Some evidence suggests that the influence of the migrant labour system has indeed been exaggerated. Migrant labourers may not be at higher risk than other groups *per se*. In one study, IJsselmuiden *et al.* (1990) found a high awareness of AIDS: 94.6 per cent had heard of AIDS, and had a relatively high use of condoms, with 32.6 per cent of the respondents claiming they used them (they did not say how often). They concluded that 'heterosexual promiscuity does not appear to be rife in the mining industry and is less than levels found in studies of other heterosexual groups' (p. 523). This echoes the claim of the Chamber of Mines, who maintains that miners play a limited role in HIV transmission. HIV prevalence

amongst STD clinic attendees at the mines stood at 8 per cent
in mid 1992, compared to a figure of 15 per cent nationally.[32]
At the mine clinic at Lesley Williams Memorial Hospital, Car-
letonville on the West Rand, however, the figure in October
1992 was 17 per cent, with approximately 11 per cent of the
total workforce presenting with an STD per annum.[33] A pilot
survey was conducted by the author at this clinic in October
1992, among the miners attending one morning session. The
most common conditions were chancroid, herpes simplex, genital lesions and warts, gonorrhoea and non-gonococcal urethritis
(NGU). Only one patient present was known to be HIV-positive, and he had a long history of recurrent STD infection. He
was from Gazankulu and stated that a local *inyanga* had failed
to cure him, and he refused to use condoms despite having
been counselled. Out of 8 miners questioned, only 1 ever used
condoms, and out of 13 questioned on where they thought they
acquired their STD infection, 7 stated their home area, while 6
stated the mine compound or nearby community. Doctors at
the clinic told me of a reputed initiation ritual at the mine
known as 'the line', in which a group of miners queue up for
the services of one or two prostitutes, and doctors at the clinic
doubt whether condoms are ever used in this kind of situation.
Such rituals could be encouraged by the need for the miners to
assert, overtly, both their heterosexuality and camaraderie in an
all-male environment.

The true extent of homosexuality in the mine hostels is
unknown, but the results of a study by Moodie (1988) would
indicate that rates of HIV transmission through homosexual
behaviour were, and continue to be, relatively low. He found
that homosexual relationships were related to social position
and tended to be monogamous rather than promiscuous. The
subordinate partner in a relationship was not allowed to ejacu-
late and sex was intercrural (involving thigh contact) rather
than penetrative. This absence of penetrative sex was also
noted by Jochelson *et al.* (1991). The debate, therefore, centres
on heterosexual activity and the extent of the use of prostitutes
and casual/regular partners by mine workers. Jochelson *et al.*
described the wide variety of relationships in which miners
engage in sexual activity, preventing the creation of a stereo-
type for the miner-sexual partner relationship. The incidence
of STDs amongst miners had increased substantially since the
mid 1970s, in part due to the apparent distrust of the management who initiated education campaigns, leading to the ignor-

ing by miners of much well-intended advice. The Jochelson study was conducted in 1988; attitudes now are probably less sceptical due to increased experience of the disease and better, more widespread education campaigns.

While evidence concerning the role of migrant mine workers in the HIV/AIDS epidemic remains inconclusive, other surveys conducted in South Africa, Namibia and Zimbabwe suggest the migrancy is indeed a considerable risk factor in HIV spread. A national KAPB study amongst hostel dwellers in South Africa revealed that approximately one third admitted to having sex with prostitutes and casual partners. Only 15 per cent claimed to consistently use condoms (Kaicener, 1993). In addition, 40 per cent believed AIDS could be cured by Western medicine. In a separate study of mine workers with STDs (DNHPD, 1993) it was found that most miners considered messages such as 'stick to one partner' as 'ludicrous'. In Kwazulu/Natal, Abdool Karim et al. (1992) tested blood samples collected in 1990 for a malaria study and reported that:

> Of the 4531 subjects for whom migrancy data were available, 9.8 per cent had changed their place of residence within the previous 12 months. The prevalence of HIV-1 infection in the latter group was 2.9 per cent, which was 3.2 (95 per cent confidence interval, 1.7-6.0) times higher than among subjects who had been living at their current address for more than a year, after adjusting for age and sex. (p. 1538)

Taking account of the gender differential, the odds ratio associated with migrancy of infection was 2.4 for women and 7.3 for men. These findings are arguably very significant, if not altogether surprising, and indicate that all migration is important, rather than just that associated with mining and institutionalised hostel dwelling. The importance of this point is emphasised when the extent of migrancy is considered: migrant labour comprised approximately 26.7 per cent of the total South African labour force in 1986, or around 2.5 million people. The figure could be as high as four million, including illegal migrants (Evian, 1993).

The influence of truck drivers should not be overlooked in the South African context. An unofficial survey conducted amongst long distance truck drivers in Johannesburg showed an HIV-1 prevalence of 25 per cent (date of survey unknown; reported in Russell, 1991, p. 24). As Peter Gould explains:

'The truck route from Malawi is now known as the Highway of Death: 92 per cent of the truck drivers visiting Durban were infected [with HIV], sleeping with prostitutes there or at stops along the way' (1993, p. 81).

The link between migrancy and diseases other than HIV/ AIDS has been demonstrated in South Africa (Packard, 1989). At Tintswalo Hospital in former Gazankulu for example, 75 per cent of TB cases seen were in ex-miners.[34] In the case of TB the relationship between migrancy and disease is complicated by the actual working conditions at the mines, which increase the chances of additional respiratory problems such as silicosis. In relation to STDs, intuition would suggest a degree of seasonality in infection rates. Seasonality has been suggested for Uganda in relation to the onset of AIDS and AIDS related complexes, due to both climatic conditions and seasonal adjustments in levels of food security (Smallman-Raynor and Cliff, 1992). Research on temporal patterns of rural STD/HIV infection rates, however, is lacking, and an early study in Boputhatswana (using data from 1987–89) failed to find any link between migrants and increased infection rates (Tshibangu, 1993). HIV prevalence at this time was very low (less than 1 per cent) and patterns of differential infection may not have been detectable due to the small number of seropositive male migrants. Repeated seasonality in rural infection rates would, however, confirm the significance of oscillatory migration in the social epidemiology of HIV/AIDS, while at the same time indicating the existence of a high risk group, namely the sexual partners (either temporary or permanent) of migrants, as well as the migrants themselves. Data from Tintswalo Hospital, along with the clinics in the hospital's catchment area, point to a temporal pattern of infection regarding STDs, as well as an upward trend in the number of cases over a period covering three-and-a-half years (Figure 3.2).

If the data are viewed for each month during 1989–91 compared to the annual mean number of cases, 'above' and 'below' average months are evident (Figure 3.3). The pattern suggests three 'above average' periods of the recording of STD incidence: March (the harvest period), June to September (the winter months and time of greatest economic stress) and December (Christmas break). The importance of migrant labour could be considerable; one estimate claims that migrancy amongst males aged 30–49 in this area is just above 60 per cent.[35]

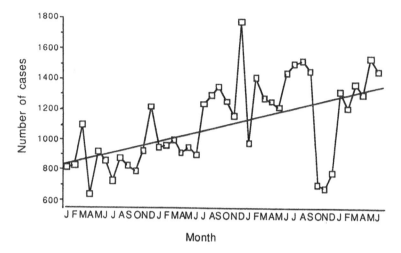

Figure 3.2. Recorded STD cases, Mhala, Gazankulu, January 1989 – June 1992

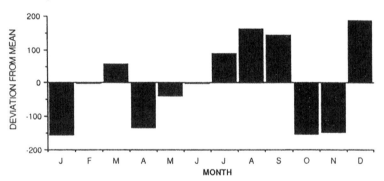

Figure 3.3. Monthly variation in STD incidence, Mhala, Gazankulu, 1989–91

Data from hospital records at Okatana R.C. Hospital, about five kilometres north of Oshakati in northern Namibia, also suggest that migration plays an important part in local HIV epidemiology (Figure 3.4).

The percentage of STD cases seen at the hospital rises disproportionately at the times of the year when migrant labourers return home – at Christmas and during the *omahangu* (millet) harvest period in autumn, around March–May. The workers would attend the out-patients department (OPD) themselves,

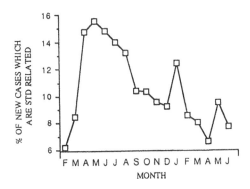

Figure 3.4. Sexually transmitted disease (STD) cases at Okatana
R.C. Hospital, Oshana, Namibia
N.B. The data relate to the period of February 1992 to June 1993
(n = 18,164), and are taken from attendance records of the out-patients
department.

possibly to be followed by their wives and girlfriends several
weeks later. This could explain the slight time-lag before diagnosis, most noticeable in the December–January period. Overall,
10.5 per cent of diagnoses were STD-related. Also, what is noticeable is the disparity in the proportion of STD cases between
March–May 1992 and March–May 1993. This drop could have
one of several explanations. As the figures represent proportions
rather than absolute numbers of cases, the figures are relative to
the number of other disease cases presented at the hospital. For
instance, a sudden influx of malaria or gastro-enteritis cases
would reduce the proportion of new STD cases reported. Seasonal changes in health could also have been exacerbated by the
1991–92 drought which may have indirectly raised the number of
STD cases (roughly twice as many as during the corresponding
period in 1993) due to the possible increased incidence of transactional sex at this time, and/or reduced body resistance to STD
infection as a result of poorer nutritional status. Drought-related
effects on food security may have marginalised many women to
the extent of relying on income from sexual favours. A third
explanation could be the improved treatment of STD cases at the
workplace, so reducing the risk of infection to the rural based
partners. During peak times of infection (notably Christmas,
periods of labour leave and school holidays in particular, as well

as small peaks such as the end of the month), intervention programmes can be stepped up, linking in with out-reach programmes, education campaigns and condom distribution. Experience shows that rarely does condom supply reach, let alone exceed, demand if integrated with an intensive education programme. This demand itself is not static and fluctuations must be recognised and accounted for in distribution.

A case in point is at the national scale in Namibia, where a pattern emerges of a movement of HIV from Windhoek to Ondangwa/Oshakati in the northern region, and return infection with migrant workers or those seeking work in Windhoek. This pattern is counter-intuitive, as the accepted pattern of HIV movement is generally southwards in southern Africa. The majority of work seekers in the Windhoek area would be based in Katutura (the former African township) and its extensions, and it is here that HIV prevalence is expected to be highest, with a figure of 7.2 per cent of a random sample of patients in a Katutura hospital reported in early 1994.[36] Secondary centres of infection are

Table 3.1. Sexual networking of HIV-positive STD patients, Onandjokwe Hospital, Oshana, Namibia

Location of sexual partner	No.	%
(Former) Owambo	5	29.4
Windhoek	4	23.5
Swakopmund	2	11.8
Kavango	1	5.9
Otjiwarongo	1	5.9
Walvis Bay	1	5.9
Don't know	3	17.6
Total	17	100.0

industrial towns such as Walvis Bay and Lüderitz, along with (presumably) the mining settlements such as Oranjemund, Arandis and Tsumeb (Figure 3.5 overleaf). Evidence from the case histories of HIV positive, sexually transmitted disease (STD) patients at Onandjokwe Lutheran Hospital near Ondangwa implicates migration as a major factor in current HIV spread. Of a sample of 277 STD patients who visited the hospital between March and July 1993, 88 (29.1 per cent) stated that the location of their sexual partner(s) within the three months previous to diagnosis, was outside of (former) Owambo, primarily in Windhoek (shown as 'per cent interaction' in Figure 3.5). This compares with the 17 (23.3 per cent of those tested) of the sample who tested HIV-positive, nine (52.9 per cent) of whom claimed to have had a sexual partner outside Owambo within the previous three months (Table 3.1).

Patients are tested for HIV according to their symptoms only; other data collected are incidental to the test, but still extremely useful. In June 1993, HIV prevalence amongst STD patients at Onandjokwe was around 20–25 per cent, but not all patients were tested,[37] so the sample is in no way representative of the sexually active adults in the area in terms of HIV prevalence. The figure can be used, though, as a comparison against other areas where sentinel surveillance occurs. Although the sample of those testing positive is very small, the difference between the HIV-negative and HIV-positive groups is still considerable and would suggest that (unprotected) sex with someone who either lives or works outside of Owambo is a relatively high risk activity with regard to HIV infection. This is consistent with many surveys which conclude that itinerants or migrant labourers are a high risk group for infection. In Zambia people consistently perceive those who travel to be at high risk, notably drivers and traders with the associated belief that multi-partnerism is a normal and accepted characteristic of this lifestyle.

The difficulty when assessing the influence of mobility and migrancy on the social epidemiology of HIV is primarily methodological. Definitions are crucial as to what constitutes 'mobility' or 'itineracy', as well as the statistical tests being used. Intuition plays a large part in many analyses, a factor which often leads to contradictory conclusions. As Serwadda *et al.* (1992, p. 988) noted in a study in Uganda:

> On univariate analysis, characteristics related to greater mobility and higher socioeconomic status (travel, education, occupation) were

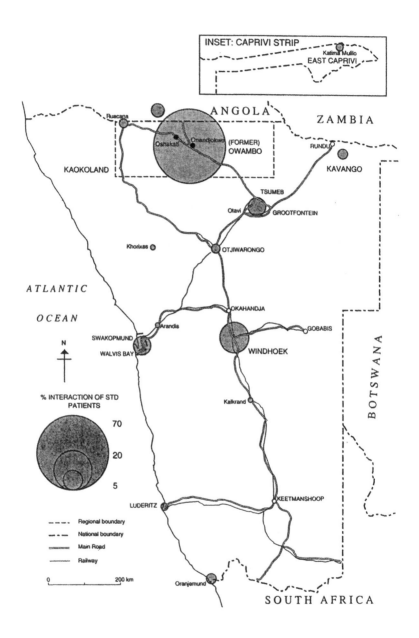

Figure 3.5 Sexual networking patterns of STD patients at Onandjokwe Lutheran Hospital, northern Namibia

associated with increased HIV levels, as were injections; however, these associations did not persist in the multivariate analysis, suggesting that these variables do not act as independent risk factors.

The reliance on statistics is possibly misleading, as the statistical divisions are fairly arbitrary and may be wholly unrelated to the perceptions and behavioural motivations of people who are either wittingly or unwittingly within high risk situations. As I have argued in Chapter 2, attributing either causal or non-causal relationships over a wide geographic area is a fairly futile exercise, as extreme variance is found at an individual scale. The distinction between what constitutes an 'independent variable' or 'proxy indicator' in terms of high risk behaviour is thus extremely blurred, especially in the case of HIV transmission. The extent of a 'high risk situation' is dependent upon both the extent of high risk behaviour and the local geography of HIV prevalence. So migrancy cannot be discounted on these terms, as migrants are clearly more likely to engage in multi-partnerism, and through their mobility are more likely to be located, either temporarily or semi-permanently, in areas of localised high HIV prevalence.

HIV and transport networks

Closely related to migrant labour is the issue of the role of transport networks in providing routeways for the spread of the virus and the determining of the pattern of localised HIV epidemiology. Evidence from the 1990 Kwazulu/Natal survey discussed above (Abdool Karim *et al.*, 1992) also supports the idea that HIV infection is associated with proximity to main roads, with HIV infection 45 per cent higher in the sectors traversed by the main trunk road compared to those away from this road. This relationship needs confirming, as clustering along the road is not wholly apparent, as shown in Figure 3.6.

Some high prevalence areas are remote from the main roads, especially those in the far north of the area adjacent to the border with Mozambique. Evidence from elsewhere in Africa, however, has clearly demonstrated an increased infection rate along main route networks (Wawer *et al.*, 1991; Barongo, 1992; Serwadda *et al.*, 1992).

The social epidemiology of HIV within the northern communal lands of Namibia (former Owambo) shows a strong relationship with the road network in the area. There were twelve reported cases of AIDS in 1989 and evidence from blood donations would suggest that HIV prevalence amongst sexually

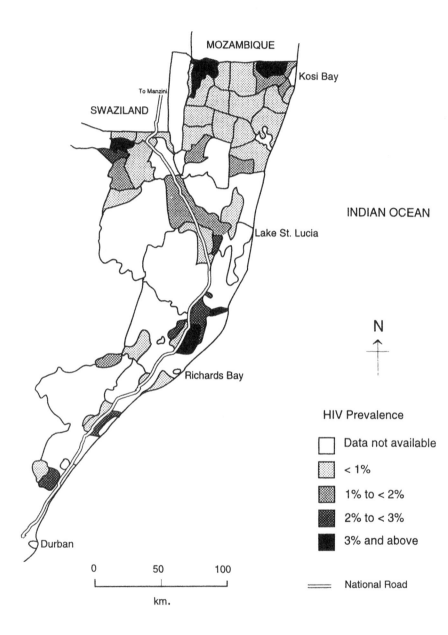

Figure 3.6 HIV infection in northern Natal, 1990 (adapted from
Abdool Karim *et al.*, 1992)

active adolescents in 1993 stood at roughly 2.8 per cent (ante-natal clinic prevalence rose from 3.6 per cent in 1992 to 14.2 per cent in 1994: Whiteside, 1995). This information was obtained from a sample of 2,228 donors, collected between August 1992 and February 1993, using a mobile donation clinic in the Oshakati/Ondangwa area. The blood was tested in Windhoek using the ELISA testing techniques. The donors were adolescents aged 16–25, as the blood collection centres were located at secondary schools and colleges. The sample shows no tendency towards self selection, which would intro-duce a large unquantifiable survey bias.[38]

The pattern of HIV spread within this area is closely con-nected to several factors: the main tarred roads through the area, traffic densities along the road network, the location of trading centres, the location of military bases and the patterns of dis-placement during the (late) 1980s. The pattern of HIV spread is northwards and westwards along the main Tsumeb-Ruacana road (Figure 3.7).

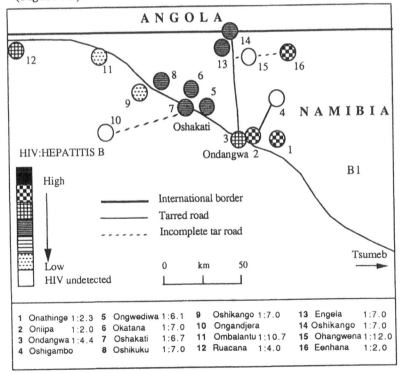

Figure 3.7 HIV clustering in northern Namibia

The pattern of spread of HIV is demonstrated by calculating the ratio between HIV and hepatitis B, a disease transmitted in early childhood in Owambo (Botha *et al.*, 1984; Kiire, 1993). The epidemiological patterns of the two epidemics are quite separate (Mertens *et al.*, 1989), and there is no correlation between hepatitis B and HIV in this sample (correlation coefficient of determination (R^2) = 0.148).[39] Using the ratio as an indicator, rather than HIV prevalence *per se*, avoids the problems presented by the nature of the data. The boundaries of the catchment areas for the blood collection centres are very ill-defined, and the samples themselves are quite small. Using the ratio also overcomes the problem of the differences in the absolute numbers of STD cases in different areas and in different age cohorts (for example the absolute number of STD cases would be higher in a sample of 25 year olds as compared to a sample of 15 year olds). The variable being tested is location, so the use of hepatitis B prevalence as a control would take into account the age cohort and extent of sexual activity variables. All blood is routinely tested for HIV, hepatitis B and syphilis. Because of these tests 12.5 per cent of samples on average have to be discarded.[40] Hepatitis B prevalence, across the whole sample, stood at 7.9 per cent, syphilis at 2.3 per cent and HIV-1 at 2.8 per cent as at February 1993. The HIV:hepatitis B ratio across the whole region during this time period was therefore 1:3.4 (n=2,228). The data on which the map is based is from donations from schools only, so standardising the age range of the samples comprising the survey. The circles on the map represent settlements where blood collection centres at schools are located.

The relationship of HIV prevalence with the main road is very evident, in that the highest HIV:hepatitis B ratios are found at the main junction (Ondangwa area) and there is a clear correlation with traffic densities, as shown in Figure 3.8. The two anomalies on the map (Eenhana and Ruacana) are related to the presence of military bases, the effects of which are discussed below. These two sites are excluded from Figure 3.8, due to their distorting effect on the relationship with traffic densities. Hepatitis B:HIV ratios (our proxy indicator of HIV clustering) are lowest on the B1 trunk road south of Ondangwa, the stretch of road with highest direct interaction with traffic from the south. This road is characterised by a series of small linear service settlements consisting of bars or *cuca* shops, garages, small shops and markets. Onathinge has a ratio of 1:2.3 (n=35), and Oniipa 1:2.0 (n=58). Oniipa is in effect a part of Ondangwa and, as

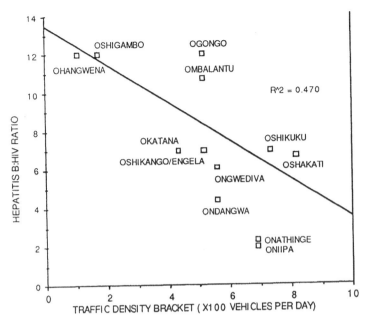

Figure 3.8. The relationship between the hepatitis B:HIV ratio at schools and local traffic densities, northern Namibia
Source: Owambo Roads Master Plan, Department of Transport, May 1992, Windhoek.

mentioned before, catchments of the blood collection centres are very difficult to determine. Beyond Ondangwa, HIV prevalence decreases farther to the north-west, and once past the major settlement of Oshakati (ratio of 1:6.7, n=>600) prevalence is relatively low. The traffic density is still high along this section of road (Ondangwa/Oshikuku) but long distance traffic is now heavily diluted with local traffic, so the absolute number of long distance vehicles is reduced; hence the relatively high ratios at Ogongo and Ombalantu. Much of the long distance traffic passes through Ondangwa and heads towards Oshikango at the border, possibly stopping at Ohangwena. Others make deliveries to the many warehouses in the Oshakati/Ondangwa area. HIV prevalence in the Oshikuku/Ogongo area is bound to continue rising rapidly in the short term. The levels of interaction with higher prevalence areas to the south-east, namely the Oshakati/Ondangwa nexus, are too significant. Between 600 to over 800 vehicles a day on average pass between Oshikuku and Oshakati.

Another area which is likely to experience rapid HIV introduction is around Ongandjera to the south-west of Oshakati. A
new tarred road is currently being built linking Ongandjera to
Oshakati and to smaller settlements such as Tsandi to the west.
This may increase traffic density to and from Oshakati (current
traffic density stands at 150 vehicles per day) and, most likely,
vehicle type, allowing more large trucks to enter this area, thus
having a possible direct influence on HIV prevalence. The road
is being constructed partly for political reasons (President
Nujoma hails from the Ongandjera area) as the traffic density in
itself does not warrant an upgrading of the existing road. Com-
muter traffic increase with the new road between Tsandi/Ongan-
djera and Oshakati may also speed up the introduction of HIV
into this area, but the real question is whether improved access
will create higher demand for goods delivered from Oshakati/
Ondangwa which themselves could have been imported from
Angola or from southern/central Namibia. The message to be
gathered here is that the development of a new road network or
link not only increases local economic opportunity, but greatly
increases the chance of the localised rapid introduction and
spread of HIV. Prevention programmes in such an area should
anticipate the health risks associated with transport developments, and target such sites as the new trading posts, truck stops
and the inevitable bars that develop. Possible large scale dam
developments on the Kunene River to the north-west in the
Kaokoveld would attract many migrant and local workers to the
sites. The inevitable increase in long distance traffic through this
northern region, as well as the influence of the construction
camps on the localised HIV epidemiology, must be taken very
seriously. HIV prevalence among the Himba of the Kaokoveld is
unknown, but a large influx of migrant workers into the area
could trigger a localised epidemic involving the workers and
local sexual networks, most probably through prostitution.

The impact of military bases on local HIV epidemiology
The most prominent anomalies in Figure 3.7 are those of Ruacana and Eenhana, which are both small military settlements.
The traffic density is not significant, but the HIV:hepatitis B
ratio is moderately high (1:4 and 1:2 respectively). This clustering of HIV at Ruacana and Eenhana is primarily due to the
military bases, where HIV prevalence amongst blood donors is
far higher than in the surrounding population (Figure 3.9).
Sexual relations between the soldiers and students at the local

secondary schools cause the HIV prevalence to be higher at the schools than expected. HIV prevalence amongst blood donors at the secondary school in Ruacana was 3.4 per cent (n=59) in 1993, while at Ombalantu secondary school, approximately 80 kilometres southwards along the main road, HIV prevalence stood at 1.7 per cent (n=174). At Eenhana, Haimbili secondary school had an HIV prevalence of 4.3 per cent and a HIV:hepatitis B ratio of 1:2 (n=46), well above the area average. This clustering is again probably due to the military base, as the settlement is relatively isolated from the main road network and has a low local traffic density of 120 vehicles per day. The four military bases in the region, of which Ondangwa and Oshakati are the largest, form the nuclei of clearly defined HIV clusters in themselves. The location of these bases reflects the strategic requirements of the South African Defence Force (SADF) during the 1970s and 1980s, to which the road network was fundamental. This also explains the high quality of the main tarred road north from Tsumeb, despite relatively low traffic volumes (Figure 3.9).

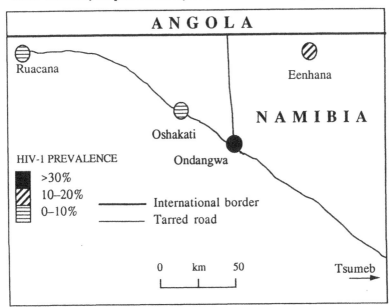

Figure 3.9. HIV prevalence at military bases, northern Namibia, 1992–93
Note: the data are derived from blood donations at the bases themselves and prevalences are as follows: Oluno, Ondangwa 33.3 per cent (n=15), Eenhana 18.2 per cent (n=22), Sector 10, Oshakati 8.8 per cent (n=57) and Ruacana 8.3 per cent (n=33).

The high HIV prevalence figures, averaging 17.2 per cent (n=127) amongst military personnel, reflect their high mobility, relative affluence and power. Moreover, many of the Namibian Defence Force (NDF) personnel now stationed there were previously PLAN (People's Liberation Army of Namibia) cadres operating out of Angola and thus at far higher risk of exposure to HIV infection. Demands for 'services' are therefore apparently being met by communities located near the bases. During the PLAN-SADF war there 'had been obvious evidence of prostitution' around these bases involving both the SADF and, to a lesser extent, personnel from the United Nations Transitional Assistance Group (UNTAG). The UNTAG was an international group of military personnel sent to Namibia to oversee the withdrawal of the SADF and provide support for the repatriation exercise.

Their departure left behind many single mothers, while many of those considered to be 'real' prostitutes left the area following demilitarisation to settle in Windhoek and the south. Perhaps more significantly 'some were described as having made a good deal of money from prostitution in the area when the SADF was present, and now had their own businesses' (Pendleton et al., 1992, p. 63). This suggests that there could be an infected pool of single mothers in the area and women who are now not engaged in prostitution. The numerical extent and geographical concentration of this group of course are very difficult to determine.

Although significant, the HIV prevalence figures among military personnel in Owambo are relatively low as compared with other surrounding countries such as Malawi, where 75 per cent of one sample were reported to be HIV positive,[41] and Zimbabwe, where in one survey the uniformed forces comprised almost 40 per cent of deaths among individual insurance policy holders (Cross and Whiteside, 1993, p. 231). However, the Owambo sample sizes are small and the figures need to be treated with caution, especially when considering possible selection biases for blood donation. Due to their high risk status, blood is no longer collected at military bases for transfusion purposes and soldiers must be regarded as a significant, mobile pool of infection, and an important target group for AIDS education and prevention.

Health structures and health seeking behaviour
The health care systems of southern Africa were wholly unprepared for the HIV/AIDS epidemic, and STDs had long been considered a widespread, but not serious, aggravation. The nature of the formal health structures did not (and still do not) allow for

an effective intervention on the scale needed to have any impact on the epidemic. Post-colonial health systems in the region are heavily biased towards the urban elites and curative rather than preventative care. Underfunding has meant that the health profiles of the populations are lamentable, even if showing signs of some improvement. Arguably, in the South African and Namibian settings, the inadequacies of the prevailing health structures prevented any possible implementation of an effective intervention at all, even if one was either available or indeed advocated. The reliance on informal health structures places many people beyond the reach of formal health sector initiatives, although with HIV/AIDS prevention these have amounted to little more than *in situ* education at clinics and hospitals, along with patchy condom and sexual health promotion programmes (Chapter 6). In fact, any glimmers of hope, in terms of treatment, are very often initiated from within the informal sector, much to the dismay of some health officials.

In both South Africa and Namibia, *apartheid* policies have had a detrimental effect on health provision for the majority of the population. The documentation on this main point is considerable and the indicators of the discrimination in health care are numerous. For example, there is a tenfold variation in the infant mortality rate between whites (6.4/1000) and blacks (66.7/1000) (Yach, 1994, p. 6). The formulation of the homeland system decentralised health care delivery to the respective states, under the control of their own budgets, which were largely determined in Pretoria. This exercise contributed to the ethos of 'blaming the victim' which the government maintained throughout in reaction to indictable health statistics from the homelands. The result was a massive underfunding of the health care structures for the majority of the population, characterised by a massive urban bias in health spending and provision; a process which continued even through such 'reforms' as the desegregation of hospitals in 1990. The resulting fragmentation of health care, both politically and geographically, led to massive imbalances in spending. The overall policy was oriented towards curative health care for whites (45 per cent of the total budget) and only marginal subsidisation of primary health care (5 per cent) for the black population, with the majority of the remainder allocated to large teaching hospitals such as Baragwanath in Soweto and King Edward VIII in Durban. Within the homelands, the development of district health care systems has often been hampered by administrative boundaries and legalities bearing no relation to the reality of geographical catchments.

A case in point is Tintswalo Hospital in former Gazankulu, bordering on one of the field areas of Mapulaneng, in former Lebowa (see Figure 2.4). Fragmentation of the administration leads to various problems, including the lack of ambulatory services, poor siting of clinics and duplication or complete absence of services. This area, along with KaNgwane, also had to absorb an influx of 100–200,000 refugees from Mozambique up until 1993 into its already overburdened health system. The understaffing of the health sector in the homelands is evident by comparing the ratios of population to medical practitioners. The figures for 1980 showed a wide variation in provision: Natal, 4,966; Transvaal, 4,405; Kwazulu, 13,286 and Lebowa, 22,360 (Botha et al., 1988, p. 849). In 1992, in Mapulaneng, Lebowa, there was one general practitioner per 16,123 people[42] and Lebowa itself arguably had the least efficient health system of all the former homelands (Packard, 1994). The inefficient and underfunded public health sector is not compensated for by the presence of an affordable private sector. Private doctors in the former Transkei, for example, are so few in number that large profits can be made in a relatively short time. In the communal lands of northern Namibia, there are only one or two private doctors serving a population of around 600,000 people. In 1993, there was only one private doctor in the Owambo region, based in Ondangwa, a situation no different to that in 1924, when only one of the 21 general practitioners in the country was in Owamboland (Gottschalk, 1988).

State restructuring of the health infrastructure in South Africa prior to the 1994 elections occurred unilaterally, without consultation with community organisations. This provision of clinics and upgrading of hospitals was viewed with extreme suspicion by many organisations such as COSATU, who anticipated that the improvements were linked to the supposedly inevitable privatisation of some health structures. Privatised institutions would remain beyond the reach of the majority population. At the previous NACOSA meeting the COSATU representative, John Gogoma retorted: 'The state is unrepresentative and cannot claim to know the health needs of the community' (NACOSA, 1992, p. 46).

The net result of inadequate public and private health structures is a substantial reliance on the household unit, followed by the informal/traditional health sector. The self reliance in terms of family and community structures for health care is admirable as well as being necessary. In the former Transkei the natal home constitutes an important resource in the management of illness. One explanation for this is that formal health care structures are inaccessible. Accessibility alone, however, certainly does not exclusively determine utilisation, as the case of contraception use testifies (Chapter 4). A complex interactive network of human resources are drawn upon: in-laws, migrant family members and children. Previous research has shown that only between 10 and 30 per cent of all illness was managed outside the family unit (Kleinman, 1978). The reliance on the informal health sector is spatially variable but prevalent in virtually all areas. Even whites in Johannesburg are known to frequent the thirty or so shops of the city-centre *inyangas*. Across South Africa, traditional medicine is used by at least 85 per cent of the black population, a figure similar to that for Swaziland (Philips, 1990) while traditional practitioner midwives deliver 60–90 per cent of the gynaecological services (Manci, 1993). There are an estimated 10,000 traditional healers in Soweto (Dauskardt, 1990).

Health seeking behaviour is dependent on a myriad of factors: the accessibility of both informal and formal services, the financial resources available, and the condition needing attention being the most fundamental. Very often, both the formal sector (the local clinic or hospital) and the informal sector (the traditional healer) will be approached through the course of treatment for a condition, and some commentators have argued that the distinction between 'Western biomedicine' and indigenous 'ethnomedicine' is naïve and simply the creation of Western anthropologists, distorting the fact that medical systems in Africa are in fact characterised by plural aetiologies. The issue is not just academic, as an understanding of the geography of health seeking behaviour, as well the geography of health, is vital if appropriate interventions are even to be attempted. To paraphrase an overused expression, the horse must *first of all* be taken to the water before making it drink. Much anecdotal evidence suggests that treatments for venereal conditions are most often provided by the traditional healer, possibly even more so than other conditions. In part, this is due to the perceived hostility of nurses and health care workers in the formal setting, as well as the strictly private and stigma-related nature of STD affliction. This, combined with misunderstandings and traditional beliefs regarding STD aetiology and treatment, discourages patients to seek help from the formal sector. The end result is a considerable under-reporting of

STD cases in the formal sector, a situation which further compli-
cates effective intervention strategies. The relative success or failure of traditional healers in the treatment of STDs is a subject of
some mystery, but in discussions with *sangomas* in central Johannesburg, they expressed every confidence in treatments. The
most popular treatment for STDs appeared to be the powder of
the crushed blister beetle (*Mylabris oculata*) mixed with water.[43]
Herbs and traditional medicines are generally used as purgatives
to remove the perceived cause of the problem, which is sometimes believed to reside in the stomach, as is the case in some
parts of Zambia. In Mapulaneng, former Lebowa, the local traditional healer mixes indigenous beliefs with Zionist Christianity,
and uses various types of teas as treatment for afflictions. The tea
is brewed in large cauldrons, then 'blessed' to instil it with heal-
ing powers. This prescription is supplemented by various forms
of psycho-spiritual support, such as singing and dancing.

Efforts towards integration of the (two) systems are ongoing
and take on a crucial importance in the light of AIDS prevention. The important issue in this context is one of the *possibility*
of effective intervention up until now. The state of integration of
the various health systems at the outset of the epidemic was
minimal, and early meetings involving AIDS education between
traditional healers and the South African Institute for Medical
Research demonstrated the gulf between the two sectors (Zazayokwe and Christie, 1990). Top down interventions, initiated at a
national scale, would only filter as far as the grass roots of formal
health care structures. It is clear that only partial reliance is
placed on these structures in terms of health seeking behaviour.
The rapidity of the spread of the virus was such that any large
scale integration of traditional health care systems with 'scientific' knowledge of the virus along with the means of its prevention, would have been a Herculean task bound to fail, due to the
lack of an historical precedent of similar immediacy. Patterns of
health seeking behaviour are deeply ingrained, especially in relation to STDs and require multifaceted approaches in changing
these patterns. Efforts to increase diagnosis and treatment of
STDs and HIV/AIDS patients have taken a considerable time to
formulate in both the formal and informal sectors. In short,
AIDS hit at a time when both the formal and informal sectors
were incapable of responding quickly to the changing sexual
health needs of the population.

Positive steps are being taken in South Africa to involve
traditional healers more closely with prevention initiatives,

despite the often huge belief gaps between the different sectors (Green *et al.*, 1995). In Lusaka, Zambia, traditional healers are being encouraged to refer patients on to the formal health care structures for treatment if AIDS is suspected, and are increasingly being targeted for technical information on the disease. Many problems still exist due to the belief gap and these have practical implications which are unavoidable. In Zambia the indigenous term for TB is *kapopo*, and is believed to be the result of sexual relations with a woman who has recently had an abortion. *Kapopo* can also relate to STDs and other unwanted afflictions across Zambia. Variations on this theme are widespread across the region. In South Africa traditional healers are now truly 'partners' in the AIDS prevention rhetoric, but how effective this rapid integration is will not be known for many years to come, and may even prove to be only a temporary union. Local health practitioners looking to utilise informal health care structures in STD and HIV prevention should do so in an open way and not look to change belief systems overnight. Experience has shown that traditional healers are more than willing to be involved in intervention initiatives and their inclusion and input is indeed vital, due to their disproportionate role in treating STDs in the community compared to other diseases (Msiska *et al.*, 1995). What is required is a change of attitudes within the formal health structures and personnel, whose arrogance in dealing with the traditional sector has prevented many positive initiatives from ever getting off the ground. The key is dialogue and an avoidance of polarising health seeking behaviour into 'us and them' – the root causes why STDs go unrecognised and untreated are very often to be found within the formal health care settings themselves.

The history of contraception and contraceptive use in both South Africa and Namibia reflects the history of *apartheid* policies, and the two are integrally linked with the divergent political ideologies of separate development and the liberation struggle. Contraceptive use estimates for 1990 are that 58 per cent of married women aged 15–49 were reportedly practising contraception in South Africa (compared to Zimbabwe, 43 per cent; Botswana, 33 per cent; Mozambique, c.33 per cent;[44] Zambia (1993), 15 per cent;[45] and Kenya, 27 per cent). Spatial differences in contraception demand relate to possible cultural and religious differences, as well as pressures to limit fertility, which are greatest in urban areas. A 1989 government survey reported contraceptive use amongst married women of 43 per cent in rural areas,

56 per cent in the Johannesburg area, and 74 per cent in Cape Town (Caldwell and Caldwell, 1993a). DepoProvera injections and the pill constituted 80 per cent of all contraceptive use. In Namibia, state policies were designed to coerce the black population into contraceptive use, very often without the consent of women, who were sometimes injected without their knowing (Lindsay, 1989). Levels of acceptance of contraception may be lower in Namibia than in South Africa, exacerbated by 'threatening husbands, physical discomfort, the church and big distances' (Ahrenson-Pandikow, 1992, p. 16).

Racial suspicion; behavioural denial
The politicisation of the epidemic has been mentioned above, but deserves particular attention as a feature which has severely hampered prevention efforts. Denial regarding the epidemic has been common to most countries to differing extents and continues today in various forms of 'otherisation' (Chapter 2). In South Africa, the issue of 'the other' being both the origin and perpetuation of the HIV/AIDS epidemic is articulated primarily along racial lines, over and above the discrimination which is related to either overt or covert homophobia, which itself is considerable. Mandela in 1992 noted that this identification of ethnicity with both the virus and political motivations is virtually inseparable:

> We do have a problem with the efforts being made by the [former] South African government, in that efforts by the government to introduce preventative measures are viewed with suspicion and as a ploy to control the population. This government does not have the credibility to convince the majority of Black South Africans to change their sexual behaviour. (NACOSA, 1992, p. 10)

The effect on prevention initiatives could only have been negative; with the epidemiological progression of two distinct patterns of infection, there arose two distinct patterns of preventative response. The political polarisation of the epidemic created the stereotypical scenario of the whites thinking that AIDS is a 'black' disease and *vice versa*. But as Mandela pointed out, could any government initiative have been taken seriously by the majority population? In the event, the initiatives were so ill-devised as to polarise the epidemic even further. Even where colour *per se* is not so much an issue, as in Namibia, early prevention initiatives (which were delayed until 1990 by the independence process) were of limited impact due to both the ethnic heterogeneity of the population and organised objection in the form of the Council of Churches. As the epidemic progresses, the issue of racial division will become less marked in terms of prevention (but possibly not in relation to epidemiology), and across the whole region churches are now generally supportive of AIDS prevention efforts. Indeed, local religious organisations are often the spearheads of prevention and caring initiatives. The promotion of condoms remains a awkward issue for the churches, but voices of dissent are now being lost in the general ground swell which acknowledges that the promotion of condom use, or at the very least the avoidance of their discouragement, is actually unavoidable. Those arguing against condoms are now in the minority and at a policy making scale rarely do they have a great influence.

In conclusion, prioritisation, which is emphasised in this chapter, is a theme that is stressed throughout the remainder of the book. The short history of the pandemic has shown that both governments and the public alike have had, in their minds, more immediate concerns of different types which negated a long term threat which the epidemic represented. What is to be realised is that the explanations regarding patterns of both infection and behavioural response are to be found through the local, regional and national contextualisation of the epidemic. AIDS prevention efforts in southern Africa have had such a minimal impact, partly as a result of their conceptually dubious origins (Chapter 2), as well as a context characterised by influences preventing the execution of an appropriate policy response: economic restructuring, poverty, other life threatening diseases, violence, political polarisation, drought, inadequate heath care provision and the lack of public leadership, which has proved so important in the United States and in Europe. Political interests and economic restrictions above all else dominated for too long, and by the time that the need for action was finally acknowledged, it was too late to change the course of the epidemic. These macro-determinants of the epidemic, which have had an almost entirely negative effect, are mediated through community and individual responses, and these are the subjects of the next two chapters.

4 The Behavioural Context of the HIV/AIDS Epidemic

The social context in which HIV is spreading is both created and interpreted by individuals. Direct questioning of individuals can reveal spatial patterns in the perceived determinants of what constitutes 'risky behaviour' in relation to HIV infection, which have been shown to be multiple sexual partners, a history of STD, particularly genital ulcer disease (GUD), of which chancroid is the most associated with HIV transmission (Chapter 1). KAPB surveys can tell us much about awareness of HIV/AIDS, knowledge of its transmission and prevention, but rarely are respondents questioned on the perceived determinants of sexual activity, be it high risk or otherwise. A political economy perspective would attribute causes to macro-processes operating beyond the bounds of community motivations or influence (Chapter 3), whereas a predominantly behavioural approach would analyse personal volition, perception, and action in relation to a risk behaviour. This section falls into the latter category while not attempting to underscore the importance of the former, although evidence does suggest that communities often seek causal explanations of behaviour which are internalised within the boundaries of the community (Butchart and Seedat, 1990). This is crucial as the possibilities for behavioural and attitudinal change at community level are recognised as the perceived determinants lie *within* the community itself. In the South African context, KAPB surveys are numerous amongst target groups such as school students (Du Toit, 1987; Mathews *et al.*, 1990; van Aswegen, 1995), mine workers (IJsselmuiden *et al.*, 1990) and urban mothers (Abdool-Karim *et al.*, 1991) but are arguably limited in both their representation and conceptual development (Skinner, 1992).

This study aims to place an attitudinal survey within its social theoretical context, and to overcome the problems inherent in those studies which are constructed in a theoretical vacuum, that is data which provide few insights into the explanation of agency action within a social context. In more simple terms, why is HIV spreading the way it is? Answering this extremely complex question in part involves the examination of the life worlds of individuals,[1] and the way in which they interpret and attempt to understand the social processes underlying sexual behaviour and the spread of HIV/AIDS (if any attempt *is* made). Taking account of socioeconomic indicators – primarily gender, age, income and status – can provide a framework for the analysis of the variety in perceptions within and between communities. Differences which are shown to be significant can attempt to illustrate not only the social epidemiology of HIV, but the reasons why attempts to stop the spread of the virus are mostly failing.

This chapter will therefore outline perceptions of the sample communities in relation to various aspects of sexual behaviour and thus the spread of HIV/AIDS, namely teenage pregnancy (adolescent sexual behaviour), the high incidence of STDs, transactional sex and prostitution. The behavioural responses to the risk of HIV transmission and the ways in which HIV/AIDS is conceptualised as a social phenomenon are discussed in the following chapter. The chi-square (X^2) test was used to identify significant relationships within the total sample of 528 respondents. Significant relationships identified by the chi-square test do not confirm any form of causation, rather the test indicates the degree to which the *observed* pattern differs from the *expected* pattern. Any relationship noted between variables is purely a case of interpretation; correlations are suggested but not statistically verified, and the direction of correlations are not given. However, the value of the test is in demonstrating relationships between determinants and socioeconomic variables, and the technique is widely used in epidemiological analyses of the HIV/AIDS pandemic.[2]

Sexual Behaviour and HIV Epidemiology

Conceptually, the perceived motivations for sexual activity are only half of the equation regarding HIV epidemiology, as the motivations for sex are only indirectly related to the factors affecting HIV transmission within that sexual activity (Figure 4.1). In the following analysis, it must be emphasised that HIV transmission is *not* under investigation, but the sociosexual con-

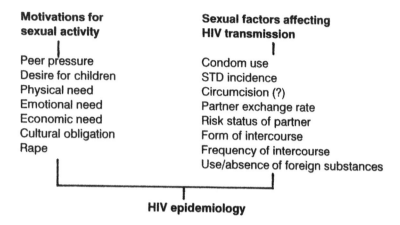

Figure 4.1. Conceptual determinants of HIV epidemiology

text in which HIV is now endemic. The use of proxy indicators for sexual behaviour is thus essential in an environment where direct experience of AIDS is very limited. The sexual framework or 'backcloth' of HIV spread is already in place; the shape of the epidemic is dependent upon it (Gould, 1993).

Teenage Pregnancy

In analysing community perceptions regarding the causation of teenage pregnancy, an outline of teenage (primarily female) sexual behaviour emerges, along with such issues as the use of, and attitudes towards, contraception, as well as the motivating factors for sexual activity. In pre-industrial societies in South Africa, as Du Toit (1987) has described, pre-marital *pregnancy*, rather than *sexual activity* was socially sanctioned against, with the penalties for pregnancy being both economic and social ostracism along rigidly determined lines.

> In the traditional black communities pre-marital sex relations were socially recognised and controlled while being regarded as moral as long as the parties conformed to the rules and norms which regulated such behaviour. (p. 562)

Pregnancy was avoided by the practice of non-penetrative sex, or intercrural/thigh sex, termed as *ukusoma* (Zulu) and *ukujami*

(Swazi). In such societies, which included the Xhosa and the Sotho, children were instructed to *juma*, rather than have penetrative sex, as the adverse social implications of pre-marital pregnancy were an adequate deterrent. Such a deterrent amongst the Zulus is *Inhwalo*: a payment of damages for pregnancy by the male or male's family. Such a fining system still exists in many areas including Kwazulu/Natal, northern Namibia and former Lebowa, where fines for illegitimate pregnancy (and also adultery) are as high as R800[3] and R700[4] respectively. With rapid urbanisation, however, such traditional sexual norms are under pressure and teenage/pre-marital pregnancy is becoming more socially acceptable, or at least less liable to cause stigmatisation. A study of high school pupils in Gauteng in 1995 found that over 80 per cent considered pre-marital sex as 'normal' (van Aswegen, 1995). It does, however, lead to many girls being forced to drop out of school, and this subject is a cause of hot policy and public debate in Zambia at the present time (Webb *et al.*, 1996). Stadler (1993) argues that the acceptance of illegitimate pregnancy in rural areas is associated with the deferral of marriage (so increasing the value of *lobola* as education can be continued), the prevention of elopement, and the enlargement of the household labour pool.

Families in urban areas are likely to be smaller (Table 2.1) and more nuclear in structure. The traditional socialisation influence of the extended family and of community elders is therefore compromised in the urban setting. This transition is most noticeable in urban areas, but social sanctions still survive to a certain extent in rural areas. For example, there is some debate over the extent of the survival of the practice of *ukusoma* in South Africa. Moodie (1988), in a somewhat different context, described the practice among male mine-hostel dwellers, but there is some doubt whether the practice survives amongst heterosexual adolescents. Du Toit (1987) argues that the practice is virtually extinct, but there is evidence that the practice survives in Kwazulu/Natal (Skinner, 1992), despite some male opposition to the practice. Some school-based AIDS education projects in Natal are attempting to encourage the practice of *ukusoma* in lieu of penetrative sex, but it is considered to be 'old fashioned' and resisted by males, who now consider full intercourse the acceptable norm.[5] Indeed, a study in Durban suggested that pre-marital pregnancy is sometimes beneficial for the girl in that her proven fertility consolidated her *lobola* value (Preston-Whyte and Zondi, 1989). In Mapulaneng, Lebowa (a Tsonga area), respondents rejected this notion as a determinant of teenage pregnancy, suggesting the cultural relativity of the importance of fertility in determining bride wealth. Different ethnic groups will place very different importance on the proving of pre-marital fertility by girls, and this specific cultural heritage will have varying degrees of influence on attitudes towards pre-marital sexual activity. The importance of fertility in Zulu culture is consistently re-emphasised. The negative association with pre-marital pregnancy is, however, universal to all my fieldwork sites, and the pregnancies themselves were numerous enough to be considered 'a problem' by the vast majority of the respondents (Table 4.1).

Table 4.1. Perceived extent of teenage pregnancy, by community

*Is teenage pregnancy a problem in the community?**		
Site	*% response 'yes'*	*% response 'no'*
Lebowa	86.0	14.0
Soweto	94.4	5.6
Natal 1 (Mpolweni)	62.8	36.4
Natal 2 (Efaye)	98.0	2.0
Oshana (Okatana)	97.0	3.0

*   The question was phrased to mean 'are teenage pregnancies *numerically significant* in the community? rather than 'are teenage pregnancies a problem *per se?*'

In Lebowa, many schoolchildren (of both sexes) expressed the desire to put off having children until after having left school, as teenage pregnancies very often mean the forced removal from school by their families. This results in a lower standard of education and inevitably a lower value of *lobola*.[6] The exact extent of teenage pregnancy can only be guessed at in this area. A survey of four schools in the nearby settlement of Acornhoek found that among the Standard 10 students, between 15–20 per cent have had children.[7] A separate estimate puts the proportion of illegitimate pregnancies at 30 per cent of the total,[8] while 26 per cent of women aged 15–34 in nearby Mhlahleni had at least one illegitimate child.[9] In Natal, a study in a Durban township found that out of 54 married mothers, 20 had given birth to children before marriage (Abdool Karim *et al.*, 1991). The prevalence of teenage pregnancy in the sample communities is unknown, but a KAPB survey of secondary school students in Mpolweni (see Chapter 5) revealed that despite the fact that all but one of the respondents are unmarried, seven (15.9 per cent) have children (age range 17–29); a low figure relative to other areas. The disparity in the perceived problem of teenage pregnancy between the two Natal communities (Table 4.1) is probably related not to the actual number or rate of teenage pregnancies *per se*, but their acceptance within the particular community. Acknowledgement is greater in Efaye, possibly because in Mpolweni teenage pregnancy is considered to have a greater stigma attached to it (being a mission community), causing some people to refuse to accept it as a local issue. Within Namibia, estimates are that more than 50 per cent of women have their first child in their teens, with the median age of one group as low as 16.3 years (UNICEF, 1990). The Namibian Ministry of Health estimated that at least 20 per cent of births in Namibian hospitals are by teenagers (Hailonga, 1993). Clearly, the rate of teenage pregnancy and thus the extent of adolescent and pre-marital sex is very high in both South Africa and Namibia.[10]

The answers to the open-ended question 'why are teenage pregnancies so common in this area?' have been grouped into the following categories: 'lack of parental care/attention, lack of information regarding pregnancy and prevention, girls need money, lack/non use of contraception, and "liking sex"'. Respondents could give more than one answer. Results are summarised in Table 4.2.

Contraception
Across the whole sample, the issue of contraception was perceived as the most important in relation to teenage pregnancy, mentioned by 26.9 per cent of the sample. Respondents described a situation where contraception is relatively inaccessible, not necessarily in a physical sense, but in that there are social barriers and it is often prohibitively expensive. In Mapulaneng, the furthest distance between a settlement and a clinic is 18 kilometres, with travelling time generally under an hour.[11] Even where

Table 4.2. Perceived determinants of teenage pregnancy

Response	Lebowa	Soweto	Natal 1	Natal 2	Oshana	Total	(%)
Lack/ non use of contraception	10.0	19.6	43.0	35.0	24.0	142	26.9
Lack of parental care	14.0	49.9	15.7	22.0	18.0	121	22.9
Lack of information	12.0	20.6	14.0	26.0	43.0	120	22.7
Lack of money for girls	18.0	14.0	12.4	2.0	2.0	53	10.0
'Like sex'	7.0	3.7	4.1	2.0	17.0	35	6.6

accessibility is *not* a problem, there are a myriad of constraints on its use: 'most of the people are unemployed, they have no money for protection' (male, 28, Natal). In Mpolweni, the mobile clinic, which visits monthly, is deemed to be totally inadequate in its primary health care delivery. Similarly in Efaye (Natal 2), which has a bi-weekly visit, the mobile clinic is considered as too inaccessible for many residents, both geographically, and in terms of the short time it spends in the village (three and a half hours), which is restricting for those who have to walk long distances. So the issue is raised of access to contraception, and it was fairly apparent that for Mpolweni residents the costs of getting to and from Pietermaritzburg (R5 round trip) to obtain contraceptives prevented people from using them: 'we haven't got clinics, and people can't afford to go to Pietermaritzburg' (female, 18). This situation will hopefully be rectified, as a new clinic was opened in Mpolweni in 1993. In Efaye, some respondents stated that they obtained condoms from the mobile clinic, and some farm

workers got them from the clinic at the nearby Noodsberg Sugar
Mill. Inaccessibility is complicated further by the lack of demand
for contraception: '... [they] don't use prevention; some don't like
it, others can't get it' (female, 24, Efaye). For most women, contraception means the DepoProvera injection, though many objections are raised to this drug: '[girls are] worried about side effects; longer menstruation and it causes weight gain' (female, 19,
Soweto). The oral contraceptive pill is also problematic for the
teenagers as they often fear that their boyfriends, and more often
their parents, will discover them. Others are unsure about the use
of the drugs: 'some girls are afraid of using prevention – they
think it is for the older people' (female, 19, Efaye). Condoms are
discussed in more detail later, in relation to both teenage pregnancy and sexually transmitted diseases.

Lack of parental care
Almost 23 per cent of respondents considered that teenage pregnancies were partly a result of the lack of parental care for the
wellbeing of the teenagers in terms of supervision. This was particularly the case in the Soweto sample, where almost half the
respondents cited this reason, compared to 14–22 per cent in the
other research sites. Why this is the case is not clear, but could
relate to a relative breakdown in intra-family communication in
the urban setting, due to the changing family structures and new
array of pressures of urban versus rural lifestyles (of which
Soweto is an extreme example). The parents are seen (by themselves in particular) to be negligent in three ways: first and most
importantly, they are not seen to be fulfilling the role of educators for their children, in terms of sexual behaviour and advice
regarding the avoidance of pregnancy; second, to be uncaring of
the children's welfare due to other domestic concerns; and third,
to be setting poor examples to the children in terms of their own
sexual behaviour. Adolescents are also seen to be deserving of
blame, and there are many indicators of inter-generational conflict within the sample communities regarding the assumption of
responsibility for the prevention of pre-marital pregnancies. In
the Lebowan field site, for example, the children were often portrayed by the adults as devious miscreants who ignore their parents and who habitually lie regarding their whereabouts and in-
tentions. A popular line used by teenagers is the expressed inten-
tion of going to school when in reality a liaison has been prear-
ranged. Night-time gatherings are also popular – but some
schoolchildren, in a focus group discussion, scorned those who

'walk at night'. In a study of sexual behaviour in neighbouring KaNgwane, of a sample of parents questioned about teenage pregnancy, 30 per cent stated that teenagers became pregnant because 'girls do not listen/want to be told what to do', while 15 per cent said that it was because 'teenagers are too free' (Radebe, 1991). In Soweto also, some respondents condemned the behaviour of adolescents: 'they are naughty, they learn about sex at school – so off they go' (male, 50); 'even though you can teach them you can never control them' (male, 75). Similarly in Natal: 'the kids think they are old enough, they take their own decisions ... and the parents don't talk to the children' (male, 19) and Okatana: 'the children don't understand and they don't want to obey their parents' commandments' (female, 24).

The onus overall appears to be with the parents, in terms of the responsibility for educating and preventing the occurrence of pre-marital pregnancies. The communication breakdown between the generations was emphasised consistently by respondents, but explanations for this breakdown were contradictory. On the one hand, sex is seen to be a cultural taboo and therefore not discussed openly, or on the other hand, that the traditional means of education through the extended family and community figureheads has itself broken down. In the KaNgwane study, 46 per cent of adult respondents emphasised the fact that teenagers were not educated about sexuality by their parents, so contributing to the high teenage pregnancy rate (Radebe, 1991). In Namibia, fully 64.7 per cent (n=102) out of the sample of students had never discussed sex with their parents: 'the teachers [should educate] – it is too difficult for parents' (female, 35). Many respondents stated that the educative role was traditionally taken by the parents and community elders, and how responsibilities have since been neglected: 'mothers traditionally gave education – better than education in schools' (female, 56). Some respondents outlined the conditions which cause there to be intra-family communication problems, such as migrant labour which separates the family both spatially and emotionally. Others simply mentioned the daily demands of subsistence: 'lack of parental control, parents don't have time for their children' (male, 46, Soweto). These quotes echo sentiments outlined in a focus group study in Katutura (Windhoek): 'some girls do not get enough love from their parents, that is why they get themselves boyfriends' and 'the relationship with our parents is so poor that we need somebody who can show us that he/she cares' (quoted in Hailonga, 1993, pp. 8–9).

Anthropological work in the eastern Transvaal has demonstrated the importance of peer group identity in rural areas and how children are socially invisible to adults to a large extent (Kotze, 1992). The ethos of children and adolescents 'fending' for themselves is a common theme in terms of information regarding sexual behaviour: 'they [the teenagers] like sex – out of their own will, so it's nobody's problem' (male, 33, Soweto). A similar notion was apparent when discussing sex education for children: 'there is no reason to teach the children sex education' (female, 39, Natal); 'no – [they] should learn for themselves' (male, 23, Soweto); and 'no, children should not be taught how to become adults' (male, 45, Soweto). Evidently, much information regarding sexual behaviour is acquired through peers and personal experience, and the example given by adults was itself condemned. The importance of peer education in AIDS prevention stems from this very strong peer information network – values and risk judgements are made in relation to the attitudes and behaviours of immediate peers, especially in the formative years of teenage and early adolescence. The perception of the behaviour of adults is also vital. In Soweto, some respondents regard alcoholism and infidelity amongst adults as being important in forming opinions of 'acceptable behaviour' amongst adolescents: 'parents set bad examples to the children ... they sleep around' (male, 24); 'our parents are also not a good example, if I see my mother is having every month another boyfriend, then I will assume that is the correct way' (quoted in Hailonga, 1993, p. 10). The important influence of parental behaviour, and that of adults generally, has also been noted in Uganda, where 23.2 per cent of a sample of primary school students mentioned 'copying adults' as a reason why teenagers engage in sexual activity (Bagarukayo et al., 1993). Central, though, to the whole issue of the formulation of adolescent sexuality and behaviour, is formal sex education.

Sex education and information provision
Knowledge regarding secondary sexual characteristics, sexual function, methods of contraception, as well as the emotional/psychological aspects of sex, are fundamental to the actual pattern of adolescent sexual behaviour and thus the prevalence of teenage pregnancy and, indirectly, HIV spread. As outlined above, the lack of information for adolescents is perceived to be crucial in determining teenage pregnancy rates. This was especially the case in the Okatana (Oshana) community (43 per cent), where access to education facilities is poorer than in South Af-

rica, and overall education and literacy rates are lower (UNDP, 1993). In both South Africa and Namibia there is no formal sex education in schools, so respondents were asked whether there should be sex education for children, and if so, who should give that education. The overwhelming majority of respondents (87.7 per cent) considered that sex education for children is appropriate. Those most suited to educate are perceived to be parents, followed by teachers and health care workers (Table 4.3).

Objection to sex education was greatest in Mpolweni (26 per cent), which is no doubt related to the mission status of the village, but those in favour were still in the majority. Similar resistance has been experienced in schools in Tanzania and Zimbabwe (which are mostly mission based) through the parent–teacher associations, who have blocked initiatives to introduce HIV/AIDS education into the national curriculum. Objection, generally, was linked to the assumption that teenagers would be encouraged to engage in sexual activity if given such education: '... some parents will object, due to culture – it may encourage sex' (male, 54, Soweto); 'no – they should know about sex after they are 21 years old' (male, 30, Soweto); 'no – they will want to experiment' (female, 42, Soweto). Some respondents do

Table 4.3. Preferred sexual health educators

Response (%)	Lebowa	Soweto	Natal 1	Natal 2	Oshana	Average
Parents	19	64	53	67	65	53.6
Teachers	10	66	24	7	24	26.2
Health care workers	28	23	23	25	17	23.2
Government	22	2	0	13	1	7.6
Community workers	1	5	3	3	7	3.8

Note: multi-answering was accepted and percentages are rounded up. Averages are simple rather than weighted.

not expect or appreciate that education is designed to reduce the incidence of unwanted pregnancies: 'no – because they will get pregnant' (female, 28, Natal); 'no – there would be a lot of orphans' (female, 23, Natal). A similar debate in Zambia concerns the role of puberty initiation ceremonies for girls, which teach the girls about sexual behaviour and the 'traditional' role of women. Due to the average age at marriage increasing and the extended time gap between initiation and marriage, it is presumed that the girl is keen to act upon what she has learned. These girls are also more attractive to males as they are officially sexually 'aware'. The practice of initiation is evidently on the decline in Zambia, but in a 1994 study of 49 secondary school girls in Lusaka, 43 per cent had undergone the ceremony (Malibata, 1994). In fact the initiation ceremonies themselves offer a useful opportunity for intervention – this institution can be utilised as a means of introducing HIV information and sexual negotiating skills. Careful participatory anthropological research is needed to investigate how HIV related information can be integrated into these ceremonies without contradicting or conflicting with existing messages.

The factor of culture as an objection to formal sex education was often raised, due to the taboo nature of the subject (which the Afrikaner administration in South Africa had consistently emphasised as a reason for not instituting sex education in school curricula), but overall it appeared that 'culture' as a stated objection was possibly replacing both the widespread embarrassment and lack of educative skills of parents. In Lebowa, a group of 60 children I spoke with had never discussed sex with their parents, and the taboo status of sex is rigidly maintained. Despite this, 83 per cent of respondents feel that there should be sex education for children, mainly from doctors and other health educators. Obviously the will is there for children to be educated, but parents do not know *how* to educate. The KaNgwane study gave similar results on perception of how to reduce the high teenage pregnancy rate, with 45 per cent responding that 'parents must teach their children about sexuality', and 20 per cent advocating sex education in schools (Radebe, 1991). The usually cited perception that culture is the main obstacle to sex education is therefore extremely simplistic. That opinion is strongest in the elderly and has to be seen as a cultural norm (possibly once applicable) which is out of touch with the needs of the young generation of today. This situation, of course, is not unique to South Africa and Namibia, but in the absence of formal education in schools, it remains a crucial obstacle to behavioural change in terms of adolescent sexual behaviour.

Some variation is apparent between the sites in terms of who are perceived to be the most appropriate educators. In Lebowa, where objection to sex education was certainly noticeable (17 per cent), health care workers were most favoured. This could be explained by the fact that a major regional hospital practising outreach work (Tintswalo, Acornhoek) is located close to the villages, despite the fact that homeland boundaries in legislation prevented such outreach work as Tintswalo Hospital is in former Gazankulu. Elsewhere, parents and teachers are seen to be the main educators, with some local variation. Teachers are seen to play the dominant role in Soweto (66 per cent), possibly because a higher percentage of children attend school than in rural areas. In Efaye (Natal 2), only 7 per cent considered teachers to be appropriate educators. Education in the Efaye community, if not from the school, will have to come from another health education body, such as the Progressive Primary Health Care Network (PPHCN).[12] In Soweto, parents are seen to play a large role in education along with teachers, but with the lack of formalised education at the present time children are only educated by sporadic visits from community nurses and such organisations as the Township AIDS Project. In Natal, plans to bring sex education into schools (the high schools in the area follow the national curriculum for state schools) will hopefully rectify the situation regarding access to information, supplementing local developments such as the new clinic in Mpolweni.

The lesson as regards information provision is that there is no set formula and that a variety of information sources provides the most appropriate set of messages. In any area different levels of trust and respect exist in relation to authority figures and institutions, and these differences should be recognised and carefully considered when analysing the possible media and key messengers. Education and information provision in relation to HIV/AIDS prevention is discussed further in Chapter 5.

Transactional sex and the monetisation of relations

An important issue which was raised, both in relation to the high incidence of teenage pregnancy and the high incidence of sexually transmitted diseases was the need for money, primarily by the girls. This direct interaction between poverty and HIV spread is so often alluded to without exploration, and there is a basic need to analyse this sociosexual phenomenon as it lies at

the heart of the epidemic, especially for the younger generation. Termed as 'transactional sex', the relationships involve
some sort of exchange in return for sexual favours, either during the course of a regular relationship, or in a more casual
liaison, which could also be defined as prostitution. In short,
sex is *commoditised*, as Dervla Murphy (1993) noted during her
travels through Tanzania:

> In Kyotera, a white fellow-guest, long involved in AIDS work else-
> where, had questioned the effectiveness of European devised educa-
> tional programmes. 'We need to remember' he said, 'that in Africa
> sex is a *commodity*. Many girls who want what they can't afford –
> clothes, cosmetics, a hair-do – will earn the money as sex workers
> and genuinely not feel ashamed. And rich men like to show their
> money by buying a variety of girls – again, as a *commodity*. It's
> another sort of mind-set about sex. (p. 161)

The theme is one of female economic dependence upon males,
and encompasses a broad spectrum of sexual relations, including
the 'sugar daddy/mummy' phenomenon, which is common across
all of southern Africa. Transactional sex exemplifies the structure-agency relationship in sexual behaviour, i.e. the distinction
between 'love and money' in sexual activity. A 'spectrum of motivation' can be devised to illustrate this relationship (Figure 4.2).

Each person who engages in sexual activity will have a set of
motivating factors. Some will be forced into an act against their
will (rape), others unwillingly through the need/want for money
(overt prostitution). Others, in the centre of the spectrum, will be

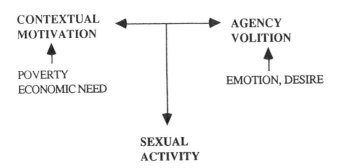

Figure 4.2. Context-agency interaction in relation to transactional sex

motivated equally by the need for money, or material contribution on one hand and genuine affection on the other. At the opposite extreme, sex will be wholly voluntary and motivated by behavioural emotions. In this case any financial or material transaction would be incidental and uninfluential as regard to the sex act itself. This conceptual scale is primarily applicable to women, but not exclusively, as the 'sugar mummy' phenomenon elsewhere has demonstrated. Anecdotal evidence from Zimbabwe, for example, indicates that adolescent girls are shunning the older men in favour of the younger boys who they consider HIV free. This process of targeting age cohorts which are perceived to be free from HIV infection inevitably results in that age cohort experiencing increased incidence rates. Certain behavioural response to HIV are actually making the virus more widespread across the age and gender spectrum.

During the course of the fieldwork and discussions with residents it became apparent that transactional sex in a South African and Namibian context is almost exclusively related to females. The phenomenon has been described in west and central/east Africa and is now a theme of growing concern regarding the development of AIDS prevention initiatives. In Nigeria, for example sexual favours are being traded in exchange for school fees (Soyinka et al., 1993), while a recent study on adolescent sexuality in Rakai, Uganda (Konde-Lulu et al., 1993), reported that

> Adolescent students frequently made the allegations that infected men use money to attract young girls for sex and that some infected men go to the extent of raping the girls. (p. 680)

and,

> Many male students strongly felt that girls engage in sexual activity for money with adults and that many girls subsequently get infected and then pass on the infection to their young boyfriends. (p. 681)

A separate study, also in south-west Uganda, in Kabale (Bagarukayo et al., 1993), asked primary school students about the motivations for sexual activity. Responses show a diversity of motivations: 'natural feeling' (quoted by 51.0 per cent of respondents); 'friends did it' (40.9 per cent); 'forced' (31.3 per cent); 'copied adults' (23.2 per cent); and 'expected rewards' (21.0 per cent). Girls were more likely to respond 'forced' and 'expect rewards', and far *less* likely to respond 'natural feeling' and 'because friends did it' than boys. The authors concluded, 'Somewhat disturbing is the rather matter of fact manner in which forced sex, rape, and money or gifts was accepted as a fact of life' (p. 13). A similar scenario is apparent in Zaire, where macro-economic changes are implicated as a determining factor: 'Although no statistics exist, observers agree that multiple partner situations, particularly those involving various forms of sexual patron–client relationships, have multiplied as economic conditions worsen' (Schoepf, 1993, p. 1402).

Transactional sex is certainly a determining factor in the field areas, and was mentioned by 10 per cent of respondents as a cause of the high incidence of teenage pregnancy, with a range of 2–18 per cent between the sites (Table 4.2). In Lebowa, it was apparent that sexual activity at an early age is associated with economic need (mentioned by 18 per cent of respondents), and that many girls quickly learn that selling favours to boys and men is one of the few, if not the only, means of gaining a bargaining advantage over them. Similarly, in the KaNgwane study, 38 per cent of adult respondents mentioned that 'girls have sex for money' in relation to teenage pregnancy (Radebe, 1991). While boys, rather than girls, seem to have a direct economic role in the villages[13] (albeit a very minor one), transactional sex is a relatively efficient method of income distribution in terms of a supply/demand perspective. When examining the incidence of teenage pregnancy, though, we can only assume that the *girls* are teenagers. If economic or material gain is the motivation for sexual liaisons, it is probable that girls would prefer older adolescents and adults, as these partnerships would no doubt prove more lucrative.[14] Respondents frequently mentioned, however, that young girls are frequently deceived with the promise of material rewards in exchange for sex. In the two Natal sites also, the economic aspect of teenage sex is demonstrated, with 11–14 per cent of respondents mentioning this factor respectively. It is expected of the boys to provide some money for the girls, even if this is a small amount: R10–R50 per month seems to be the standard. This is in no way classed as prostitution, but just one of the unwritten rules of a sexual relationship. Many teenage girls explicitly stated that if their boyfriend did not provide them with money or small gifts on a regular basis, then they would 'love somebody else'. The economic climate in the Natal area was also perceived to have an impact: 'girls go for the boys with most money' (female, 17); 'women sleep with anyone ...

because there is unemployment' (female, 27); 'unemployment and they sleep with anybody to get money' (male, 24); 'sometimes they are trying to get money, because blacks ... they have got no money' (female, 23). The point is that the nature and extent of transactional sex will respond to variations in economic stress and vulnerability in this context is directly related to poverty.

In the urban setting of Soweto, 14 per cent of respondents mentioned the need for money as a cause of teenage pregnancies. A study in 1990 of Soweto households found a negative correlation between a daughter being pregnant and per capita income, indicating an economic determinant of adolescent sexual activity (Turton and Chalmers, 1990). It was repeatedly pointed out to me that most sexual relations have some sort of transaction involved – money, food, drinks, favours, clothing – and that girls evidently expect some sort of payment throughout the course of a relationship. Again, this is not to be classed as prostitution, more a socially sanctioned way of money distribution through the youth. There are more wage earning opportunities for males than for females, and this is one way of rectifying the situation for the females. The males accept this as a fact of life and many schoolchildren are involved in these sort of exchanges once becoming sexually active. The behavioural aspect of sexual enjoyment is certainly associated with economic gain for the girls and mostly the latter is a pleasant concomitant of the former: 'parents don't have the means to maintain them ... [girls] resort to guys who could provide them with clothing, food' (male, 17); 'some girls need improvements in life – take on boyfriends for favours' (male, 54); 'girls want money, guys just want sex' (male, 16); 'girls are after money – they go out with guys with cars' (male, 16); 'both parties are not satisfied ... greedy; others give credit cards: R50' (female, 21).

In the Oshakati area, among the students surveyed, transactional sex on the whole is an accepted reality. To the question: 'Is it usual for a boy to give his girlfriend gifts and money?' 67.6 per cent (n=102) of respondents said yes, 30.4 per cent said no, and one respondent did not answer. Questioned on how much a boy is expected to give a girl, responses ranged from R2–R350 per month (about £0.40 to £70). Most respondents who answered explicitly, claimed that R20–R100 (£4–£20) per month was the norm. The range of amounts expected is surprising, and many respondents claimed that the amount is agreed before any sexual activity takes place. Those who are working are expected to give more than students, while men with jobs are keenly sought after by the schoolgirls. This proved to be a cause of resentment amongst the boys at one school. The girls have relationships with boys who are on average three years older than themselves, and money in part explains this; 'student – R5 per month; worker – R50 per month' (male, 25), 'if he is employed he can give her R100 per month' (female 16), 'he can give 2 soaps and R10 per month' (male, 21), 'many partners ... because of money ... parents don't give children enough ... boys give money, R20–R50 per round' (female, 19). In Katutura, the situation is no different: 'the reasons why teenage pregnancy is so high, is [sic] because schoolgirls go out with working men, because they have cars and money to give them' (quoted in Hailonga, 1993). There is latent opposition to this informal institution as it is seen by some to encourage prostitution: 'no, she will get used to the money until she starts selling herself' (female, 20, Okatana). The wider issues involved are quite serious: gender relations and women's economic dependence on men, which evidently starts at an early age, and continues right through life. Men are obviously aware of their strong bargaining position in relation to sexual activity and exploit this dependence relationship: '... yes, particularly here in Africa – we do it [give money and gifts] just for making girls believe that a man loves them, though they are just deluding themselves to think that a man loves them' (male, 27, Ongandjera).

The important question in relation to transactional sex is whether transactional sex affects the actual amount of sexual activity in any community, or simply affects the choice of partners, so leading to the emergence of core groups. There is some evidence for the latter argument, from research in Burundi (Sokal et al., 1993) and amongst factory workers in Harare, as Bassett (1993, p. 10) noted that in order to save money, 'some men are now forgoing girlfriends because of expense and are opting for paid single sex encounters'. Serwadda et al. (1992) argue that because of the difficulty in quantifying and demonstrating statistically the relationships between transactional sex and other risk factors, it can only be used as an intermediate or proxy measure for high risk behaviour. Evidence from the central African AIDS belt indicates that in the initial stages of the epidemic, the (urban) elite classes were most vulnerable, due, in part, to greater sexual freedom through increased purchasing power. This distinction is difficult to address, and transactional sex, as a phenomenon, merges with covert and overt prostitution in terms of classification. Prostitution is discussed in relation to sexually transmitted diseases, but the separation of the two entities is one of degree rather than type.

Emotional aspects of adolescent sexual behaviour account for only 6.6 per cent of responses in relation to teenage pregnancy ('Like sex' in Table 4.2). This figure may be surprisingly low, but it is indicative of the monetisation, or commercialisation of sexual activity, which brings the prospect of material reward into possible conflict with emotional feelings. The love/money distinction cannot be examined in isolation from the integral complexity of the acting determinants or conceptually removed from other processes operating at a local scale:

> Parents pointed to poverty, over-crowding, lack of recreational and educational facilities and to the fact that many mothers have to work in rural areas when asked why teenage pregnancies occur so frequently. (Preston-Whyte and Zondi, 1989, p. 60)

Focus group discussions with school students in the Oshakati area revealed divided opinion amongst students regarding the role of material exchange within relationships, with many insisting that sexual activity was solely motivated by emotional aspects. A similar situation was evident in the Katutura study (Hailonga, 1993). All discussants agreed, however, that wealthier men 'get more girlfriends'. This attraction of status is no doubt universal, but in the southern African context, exchange and sexual activity seem to be so inextricably linked as to be concomitants of each other. The links between sexual and economic independence for women are incredibly complicated, but there is no doubt that a certain degree of adolescent sexual activity is a direct result of the financial dependence of women on men. This factor of course will vary at an individual scale (Figure 4.2). Micro-scale analyses can aid in the categorisation of those who are most vulnerable and economically marginalised (and how this changes over time) in relation to HIV infection as well as to teenage pregnancy, as the risk factors are essentially the same. The pattern of HIV epidemiology in sub-Saharan Africa repeatedly shows peak prevalence in women in the low to mid twenties, with men in their late twenties and early thirties. Infection rates are growing fastest in young women, including teenage girls, reflecting both the 'sugar daddy' phenomenon, the physiological vulnerability to infection of younger women, and the sexual status of older, rather than younger men, in terms of relationships with teenage girls. There is a widespread belief in Namibia, for example, that only working men can impregnate schoolgirls (Hailonga, 1993). President Nujoma even went as far as threatening in early 1994 to introduce a law forcing men to marry teenagers whom they had made pregnant. The importance of this partnering trend is realised when both research and anecdotal evidence shows that condom use in these relationships is lower than in those involving schoolgirls and schoolboys (Soyinka et al., 1993).

A situation which could encourage a high rate of teenage pregnancy is one where recreation facilities are lacking. In former Lebowa, the PPHCN has taken to installing volleyball nets in villages, as a means of encouraging physical activity in lieu of sexual curiosity and experimentation, as well as an effort in sports education. Youngsters were already involved in football and netball, so the volleyball may only act as a temporary distraction. Similar sentiments were expressed in Natal by respondents regarding lack of recreational facilities and the link with teenage pregnancy: 'they have got no sports' (female, 20). The complexity of the situation demands an integrated approach, in which sports facilities can only *supplement* more immediate demands (Chapter 6).

Gender, age and income differentials in perception of teenage pregnancy
The analysis of perceived determinants presented above gives the generalised picture, but there is certainly no homogeneity, either between the sites or along the lines of gender, age or income. The importance of heterogeneity is realised when planning prevention programmes and indeed in predicting community responses. The targeting of those who are most vulnerable is still a crucial aspect of sexual health education. Between the field sites, great gender variation is shown in apportioning causation to the different determinants (Table 4.4 overleaf).

Overall, females were more likely to mention the lack of contraception than males in relation to teenage pregnancy, especially in Soweto and Efaye (Natal 2) ($p<0.05$), indicating an overall greater awareness of contraception than among males. This could relate to the targeting of education programmes through the formal health sector and the perceived responsibility which women take, or are assumed to take, for the obtaining and use of contraception. Males were more likely to men-

222

Table 4.4. Gender differentials in the perceived determinants of teenage pregnancy

Site	Lack parental care (%)		Lack of information (%)		Girls need money (%)		No contraception (%)		Like sex (%)	
	F	M	F	M	F	M	F	M	F	M
Lebowa	20.3	4.9	1.7	26.8	22.0	12.2	10.2	9.8	8.5	4.9
Soweto	46.0	43.2	15.9	27.3	11.1	18.2	25.4	11.4	4.8	2.3
Natal 1	16.7	14.3	8.3	22.4	11.1	12.2	48.6	34.7	1.4	8.2
Natal 2	16.1	31.6	19.4	36.8	4.8	2.6	43.5	21.1	1.6	2.6
Oshana	16.7	20.0	36.7	52.5	3.3	0.0	23.3	25.0	18.3	15.0

F = female, M = male

tion the lack of information as a determinant ($p<0.001$), illustrating the gender bias in access to information provision and flow (Chapter 5). Perceptions also altered according to age cohorts (Figure 4.3). The younger age groups, for example, are more likely to mention a number of issues: 'like sex' ($p<0.05$); lack of contraception use ($p<0.001$); and, although not very significant, the lack of information (p0.073). The older respondents were more likely to mention the lack of parental care (which includes the category of parents not talking to their children) to a significant degree ($p<0.05$), especially those in the age band of where parental responsibility is most relevant. On analysis, it seems that teenagers give almost equal weight to each of the categories, while points of view diverge amongst the older groups, especially those in late-middle age. It is probably no surprise that younger groups relate to the behavioural aspects of sex, along with issues surrounding contraception and the lack of information provision, as they are the causes which have greatest relevance to adolescents experiencing sexual

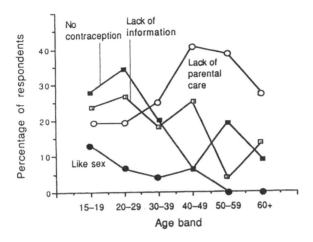

Figure 4.3. Perceived causes of teenage pregnancy by age

development and maturation. Parents are obviously aware of the role that they and their peers are sanctioned to take by society (although this issue of 'who should educate?' is surprisingly complex), but do admit that the parental body is not fulfilling the role of educator. Younger people would not be aware of this role of the parents to the same degree, as their primary information sources would be peer groups and targeted education campaigns, which would supplement personal experience. There was no relationship between age group and the response of 'girls/women need money', presumably because female economic dependence on men is something relevant to all age groups to similar extents, and is an overall characteristic of patrilineal societies. In other words, *everybody* is aware of the 'sugar mummy/daddy' phenomenon and the reasons for its existence.

Considering marital status, unmarried people are more likely to mention the lack of information (p<0.05) and the lack of contraception (p<0.001) than those who are married. The issue of information would, in part, be explained by age factors, but the strong association with contraception would relate to a possibly moralistic stance of those married, that is deliberately not mentioning it as teenagers 'should not be sexually active' at all. Reports emphasise that many parents are genuinely unaware that their children are sexually active anyway, as is the case in many

societies. Alternatively, it could indicate a genuine low awareness
of extra-marital or indeed nuptial contraceptive use, for whatever
reason. Those who are married again emphasise the issue of lack
of parental care ($p < 0.05$), indicating the awareness, but not fulfil-
ment, of the educative role.

Perceptions of Sexually Transmitted Diseases (STDs)

As HIV is an STD, and very often closely linked to other STDs
such as chancroid, community perceptions of STDs are examined
in terms of their prevalence. In analysing the perceived determinants of the high incidence of STDs, the sexual behaviour of a
slightly different age cohort is under study, that is those in their
twenties and thirties, as these are the cohorts showing peak STD
prevalence. Medical records from Tintswalo Hospital in Acornhoek show an average mean age for STD patients of 28.7, with
males 30.1 and females 27.3 (Figure 4.4).

The records at Tintswalo also show that approximately 10 per
cent of all out-patients present with an STD, a similar figure to
that in the Oshakati area. The mean ages were 27.3 for women
and 30.1 for men. In Okatana, the most common genital infections are gonorrhoea, chlamydia, chancroid, syphilis and cervisi-
tis. Over a 17 month period at Okatana Roman Catholic Hospital, 1,911 new cases of STDs were diagnosed. Syphilis prevalence
amongst blood donors for the north-west Owambo region in
February 1993 stood at 2.3 per cent. Statistics of STD prevalence

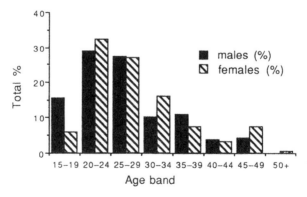

Figure 4.4. Age distribution of STD cases at Tintswalo Hospital,
Acornhoek, June–October, 1992

in rural Natal are difficult to obtain, but figures from the Noodsberg Sugar Mill, adjacent to Efaye, show an incidence of 10.6
new cases per month. Over a 13 month period up to March 1993,
138 cases were reported (mainly chancroid, urethritis and non-
gonoccocal urethritis) out of a workforce of less than 1,000.[15]
STDs are a crucial aspect of HIV epidemiology. They indicate
patterns of existing sexual activity and hint at future HIV spread.
STD infection is a known risk factor and increases the chance of
HIV infection by up to a factor of five per sexual act (Laga *et al.*,
1991; Chapter 1). An STD control programme is therefore also a
direct HIV control programme.

The question responses again are open-ended and the results
are strikingly similar between the communities, showing the
strong influence of common social forces (Table 4.5).

Table 4.5. Perceived determinants of the high incidence of
sexually transmitted diseases

Response (%)	Lebowa	Soweto	Natal 1	Natal 2	Oshana	Ave.(%)
Many partners/ promiscuity	40.0	58.9	43.0	59.0	63.0	52.8
Women need money	22.0	13.1	43.8	42.0	17.0	27.6
'Like sex'	6.0	7.5	8.3	13.0	46.0	16.2
Lack of information	4.0	10.3	16.5	13.0	5.0	9.8
Lack of contraceptive use	3.02	5.2	4.1	6.0	5.0	8.1

Uncovering the perceived reasons why STDs are so common
in the community often reveals hidden prejudices. For example,
9.1 per cent of respondents in Mpolweni mentioned the mixing

of races as the main reason. Of the respondents questioned, about half (52.8 per cent) simply felt that promiscuity is the cause of the high STD rate. Females were more likely than males to mention promiscuity in this regard (p<0.05). The explanation of this is not clear; it could reflect a non-judgmental shared opinion, a moralistic statement on other women, or be a subtle reference to the behaviour of men. This reference to promiscuity does not imply any causation, but indicates the extent of 'multipartnerism' in these communities. The debate over the extent of promiscuity in African societies has been lively, but so often imbued with either racism or academic political correctness that the reality of the situation is so often misconstrued and invalidated, as Feldman (1991) noted:

> For those African societies where multipartnering behaviour and sex-positive attitudes are common, applying the pejorative label 'promiscuous' is an ethnocentric affront; defending those societies from that label by pretending that these behaviours and attitudes either do not exist, or exist only as a neo-colonial pathology, is a comparable affront. (p. 784)

In southern Africa, reliable data on the extent and nature of sexual activity are scarce, with anecdotal evidence so often informing opinion without quantification. Respondents' comments indicate the community perception of multipartnering behaviour: 'promiscuity; even though they have one relationship at a time, they may have more than six relationships in a year' (male, 46, Soweto); 'people don't stick to one partner, they sleep with anyone, Xhosa, Zulu, Sotho, she doesn't bother what ethnic group' (female, 25, Soweto); 'it is Zulu culture to have many partners' (female, 24, Natal); 'girls have many partners inside and outside the village' (male, 23, Natal). The perception in Soweto was that sexual activity was certainly related to social status, and for the males an important expression of their masculinity, possibly heightened in an environment where other opportunities for status display and competition are limited: 'sex is viewed as something for fun ... also fame; if they sleep around they become famous' (male, 23). The more sinister side of sexual conquest to prove status is most noticeable in Soweto also, where the incidence of rape is estimated to be in the region of 2,000 per month, and more than half of the rape victims are below the age of 16 (Fleming, 1994). This phenomenon, known as 'jackrolling', involves the gang rape of young girls, and is reportedly on the increase in the township and a considerable problem in terms of HIV transmission. Alcohol and drug abuse have also been linked to HIV transmission in that (unsafe) sexual activity is increased by their use. This was mentioned by respondents but did not seem to be an overriding issue: 'girls are bitches – when they get drunk they will sleep with anybody' (female, 38, Natal); 'people sleep with anyone, they eat some food ... like peanuts and cheese, and they get excited' (female, 51, Natal).

Substantiating claims of widespread multi-partnerism is a sensitive issue to address, not only in terms of methodology but also politically. The immediacy of the epidemic requires that these questions are asked in the most objective, value-free manner possible. A KAPB survey was conducted in Mpolweni, Natal, with a group of secondary school students covering issues relevant to HIV epidemiology (the survey is discussed in more detail in Chapter 5). The 45 respondents were aged 17–29 and were all students at the school, either in Standards 9 or 10. The respondents were questioned on the extent of their sexual activity (Figures 4.5 and 4.6).

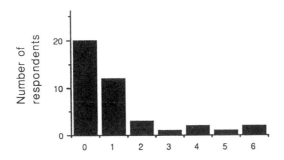

Figure 4.5. Number of sexual partners in past three months, secondary school students, Mpolweni Mission, Natal

The results show that 52.2 per cent of the sample had been sexually active (with 21.9 per cent having two or more partners) in the previous three months. The sexual profile of these adolescents and young adults is arguably no different from that of any Western society (Table 4.6). In the same survey, 42.2 per cent of the sample agreed with the statement that 'it is OK for teenagers to have sex', while 31.1 per cent disagreed and 26.7 per cent were not sure.

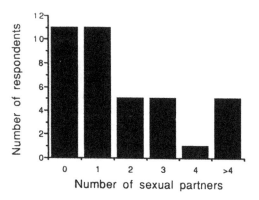

Figure 4.6. Number of sexual partners in past twelve months, secondary school students, Mpolweni Mission, Natal

Table 4.6. Extent of sexual relations amongst secondary school students, Mpolweni, Natal

Nature of present sexual relationship	No.	%
No sexual experience	5	11.1
Presently sexually inactive	10	22.2
No regular sexual partner, but sexually active	2	4.4
One regular sex partner	20	44.4
More than one sex partner	7	15.6
No answer	1	2.2
Total	45	100

Two respondents (4.4 per cent) have only had homosexual relations.

In Okatana, 63 per cent of respondents considered promiscuity as the most important reason for the high incidence of STDs: 'running from one to many partners' as one female, aged 51 put it. Conversely, the KAPB survey of students around Oshakati revealed a strong rejection of promiscuity as a form of behaviour. To the question: 'Is it OK for a boy to have many girlfriends?' 87 (85.3 per cent) said no, only 14 (13.7 per cent) respondents said yes, and 1 (1 per cent) did not know. To the question 'Is it OK for a girl to have many boyfriends?': 94 (92.2 per cent) said no, only 6 (6 per cent) said yes, and 2 (2 per cent) did not know. The high stigma attached to promiscuous behaviour indicates an associated high stigma attached to STDs, and anecdotal evidence suggests that STDs are under-reported in the area because of this stigma: 'some people shy from getting STDs treated at hospital, though they know they are infected' (male, 32). To the question of acceptance of many partners, one respondent hinted at the impact of AIDS on attitudes towards promiscuity: 'no, this current situation does not permit us to do so' (male, 28).

When pressed on why people have many partners, a variety of responses were given: need for money (27.6 per cent), enjoyment of sex (16.2 per cent) and immorality (less than 5 per cent). An Okatana respondent noted the demographic imbalance in the area; 'men have many partners ... there are more women than men' (female, 25) and she claimed that some men justified their promiscuous behaviour by quoting this imbalance.[16] Also in Okatana, one respondent noted the high population density in the area which somehow facilitates sexual promiscuity; 'men and women are close together, and most of them like sex' (female, 40), while others seemed to accuse men exclusively; 'men have many partners, men like sex' (male, 20). So promiscuity is perceived to be the outcome of a combination of behavioural and contextual/economic factors. Money and material goods may be a usual part of sexual activity but the question has to be of how much importance is placed on this exchange within the relationships. Sexual activity cannot be exclusively assumed to be an economic coping mechanism, as the behavioural component of motivation is perceived to be considerable. In other words, even if living standards were markedly improved, promiscuity with the resultant high rate of STDs would still be prevalent (possibly to a lesser extent), so implicating other socio-behavioural factors.

Unmarried respondents were more likely to mention the enjoyment of sex (p<0.01) and the issue of girls/women needing money (p<0.005) in relation to the high incidence of STDs. This

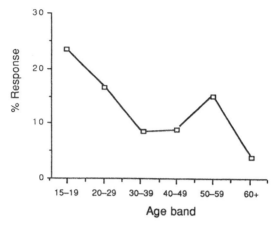

Figure 4.7. Behavioural determinants of the high incidence of STDs, by age

is not surprising, as single people are more likely to be both promiscuous, or aware of promiscuous peers, and/or involved in relationships involving transactional sex. This is not to say that transactional sex does not involve those either married or divorced; but it may be more indiscreet in those who are single. The attributed importance of behavioural factors also varies according to age (Figure 4.7).

As in relation to teenage pregnancy, the point is echoed by the youth of the perceived importance of the behavioural aspects of sexual activity, and are more likely to mention 'like sex' than the older groups (p<0.05). A study among women in Dar es Salaam confirmed that the tendency to have multiple sexual partners decreases with age and with education (Kapiga *et al.*, 1993). There was no significant relationship between the other determinants of STD incidence and age group, although younger people *tended* to be more aware of the issue of money and of promiscuity.

Prostitution

The large issue of transactional sex has been discussed in relation to teenage pregnancy, but is equally applicable to the spread of STDs, and conditions of poverty cannot be removed from their social epidemiology. A related issue is that of prostitution, which is widely implicated in the spread of STDs including HIV. A widespread review of sexual behaviour across Africa found that 0.2–13 per cent of adults had engaged in commercial sex in the previous twelve months (Carael *et al.*, 1991). Respondents in this study were asked about the social causes of prostitution, which also had the effect of uncovering social attitudes towards prostitutes as a marginalised group, and their perceived role in the spread of STDs and HIV/AIDS (Table 4.7).

Table 4.7. Perceived determinants of prostitution

Response (%)	Lebowa	Soweto	Natal 1	Natal 2	Oshana	Ave. (%)
Poverty/need money	50.0	94.4	94.2	92.0	81.0	82.3
'Like sex'	8.0	13.1	15.8	3.0	18.0	11.6
Poor family background	2.0	13.1	11.6	0.0	0.0	5.3
Lack of education	0.0	6.5	5.8	0.0	0.0	2.5
Not satisfied with one partner	8.0	1.9	0.0	0.0	0.0	2.0
Want to spread diseases	0.0	0.0	0.0	0.0	4.0	0.8

The principal cause of prostitution is undeniably poverty, compounded by a combination of factors such as poor education (and education opportunities), and a family background characterised by neglect and poor socialisation. Again, emphasis must be placed on the multi-causal nature of a behavioural sexual category, as other determinants operate over and above those simply economic: 'Investigation of the motivations for sex work should include the subjective feelings of persons, their economic need, the development of their sexual identity, and situations of possible physical coercion or social pressure' (Parker *et al.*, 1991, p. 83).

With prostitution at mine compounds, local women are most often forced into prostitution for financial reasons (unemployment), often caused by the breakdown of a marriage or relationship where the woman was economically dependent upon her partner (Jochelson *et al.*, 1991). Overall, respondents from the survey stressed economic motivations (82.3 per cent) for entering into prostitution, a figure echoed by a survey of prostitutes in Cameroon, where 86.4 per cent of those questioned stated that they entered prostitution for financial reasons (Nyudzewira *et al.*, 1993). In Lebowa, economic causes of prostitution were linked in with inadequate remittances from migrant husbands by some female respondents, along with the lack of labour opportunities for women. One respondent (a 28 year old woman teacher) replied, 'prostitution is the most important employment [for women]'. Some women seek sexual partners for emotional reasons, due to the absence of the husbands, but overall poverty was forcing most of these women into prostitution. But behavioural motivation should not be underestimated – 16 per cent of respondents gave strictly behavioural responses (not satisfied with one partner/like sex/natural). It is possible that behavioural reasons are cited by others who themselves do not face such severe economic hardship – the statement then becomes one of moralist indictment. In reality, of course, a complex interaction of factors would lead a woman into sexual activity for material or economic gain.

In Soweto, the majority (81 per cent) of the respondents do not know of any prostitutes in the community, and it soon became apparent that the term 'prostitute' has a precise meaning. A prostitute is a woman who sells herself for a living, i.e. as a 'professional', but this activity was mainly associated with the district of Hillbrow in Johannesburg. One male respondent even went so far as to say the he knew a certain woman, and that she was a prostitute 'because she lives in Hillbrow'. I was told on several occasions that there are no prostitutes in Soweto, as 'all the escort agencies are in Hillbrow' (there are in fact some in Joubert Park and in central Johannesburg). The common forms of sexual exchange which take place in Soweto are not perceived to be prostitution at all, and being a professional in the trade carries with it a large stigma: 'prostitutes hide themselves for fear of being killed' (male, 50). The distinction was also made between wants and needs, and some prostitutes were said to be 'greedy', implicating that income was often surplus to essential requirements: 'money, these girls are in love with money, they don't care about themselves' (male, 25). Even so, 13.1 per cent claimed that these women are motivated because they 'like sex' and there is no doubt that there is a behavioural component for some prostitutes, which could be related to the desire for independence, but again this has to be seen in the wider context of poverty and economic coping. One respondent even placed emphasis on the role of economic sanctions in creating the situation where women are driven to prostitution.

In the Soweto context, it is possible to classify commercial sex work/prostitution into three broad categories. The existence of the second category became apparent following many discussions with community residents on the issue of poverty and sex work.

Sexual exchange involving adolescent girls. Schoolgirls may take on a 'sugar daddy' who buys them presents, particularly clothes. Boyfriends of the same age are also expected to provide some sort of 'payment'. As a result girls are attracted to wealth and status.

Sexual exchange involving women who may be single parents or divorced. Such women are often uneducated, having been forced to leave school, and are unable to find employment. Migrants from rural areas often find themselves forced into such a situation where domestic income is either nonexistent or insufficient. In these cases, the women may have a small ring of boyfriends who provide for her, for example food, clothing and school fees. This would not be considered as prostitution and is fundamentally an economic coping mechanism which may be used only in the short term, or during periods of domestic instability.

Sexual activity related to a woman who would classify herself as a prostitute, drawn into the lifestyle often heavily influenced by peer pressure. These women are perceived to be professionals, often linked with escort agencies, and almost exclusively associated with the district of Hillbrow.

In the Natal context, anecdotal evidence suggests that a core of prostitutes exists in Mpolweni, who work both within the community and at nearby truck stops. Some itinerant workers constructing the new clinic in the village were reputedly visited at night by a small group of prostitutes while camping near the site. One respondent claimed that there are over 100 prostitutes in Mpolweni, whose clientele mainly consists of truck drivers who stop at Pietermaritzburg. As in the Soweto setting, the Western concept of prostitution is very blurred in these rural communities, as the variety of commercial sex work forms a long spectrum from prostitutes in urban areas who have 15–20 clients per night, to a schoolgirl who expects some material reward from her boyfriend. In Efaye, there are known prostitutes who 'trade' both inside and outside of the community. Prostitutes there charge R20 and one respondent claimed that they would earn around R200 per month. Another respondent stated that she knows some prostitutes in Durban who earn up to R1,000 per night, where the going rate is R50 for 15 minutes. In rural New Hanover, activity is more modest but can still be quite organised. A security guard at Noodsberg Sugar Mill described the influx of prostitutes into the mill compound on pay days (a similar situation had been described in the Transvaal by Jochelson et al., 1991). He added that activity had declined in recent years, without offering any explanation why.

In Okatana, perceptions of prostitution also generally identify economic need as the main causal agent, but the definition of prostitution in this context seems to be more related to the number of partners a woman may have rather than whether there is a money or material exchange taking place. Prostitutes themselves are perceived to be 'malicious' by a small minority of the sample, in that they are prostitutes *because* they want to spread STDs, through some sort of revenge motive. The association of prostitution and disease is fairly common, along with the perception that males are vulnerable to infection through contact with prostitutes, as a quote from a Natal man demonstrates: 'prostitution is wrong and should never be legalised. It is mostly males who later become victims because of the diseases they get from prostitutes'.[17] Overall in Okatana, however, money is perceived to be the driving factor, although 18 per cent thought that behavioural motivations were dominant: 'they want to parasite the men' (male, 20); 'some want money ... others get drunk and become prostitutes, they don't know what they are doing' (female, 27); 'earn some money, R300–400 per round' (female, 38); 'poverty – sometimes related to pregnancy and rejection from parents' (female, 25). A camp near the 'location' at Okatana housing construction workers building a water pipe was proving a strong magnet for some local women, and one female respondent was pregnant with a child supposedly fathered by one of the camp workers. Another woman staying at the camp had been treated for an STD at the hospital. There was no overt prostitution at Okatana and this is explained by the fact that most of the known prostitutes operate in nearby Oshakati.

Information and the Provision of Health Services

The aspect of lack of information was mentioned by 9.8 per cent of respondents and the issues are fundamentally similar to those involving the teenage pregnancy rate. This point is very pertinent, as STDs are likely to be underrepresented in official medical records, and to remain undiagnosed by the patients themselves. Women very often fail to recognise the symptoms of STDs, and even when they do there is a marked reluctance to get them treated in the formal health care setting. The lack of information on the diseases is translated into attitudes and behaviour. In Lebowa, I was told by one respondent that 'white people cannot cure it [STDs] at the hospital, they give you pills, after a few days you feel well, then, after about four months, it comes back' and 'injections they get cause diseases' (male, 17, Natal). Problems with STD treatment due to lay misconceptions are also evident in Zambia, where chancroid treatment is often not completed due to the delay before any visible recovery of the lesion(s) is evident.[18] Misconceptions are not only related to the aetiology and treatment of STDs: 'All 39 women in a survey in three villages in Mhala believed that TB is caused by one of three forms of improper sexual practices after the death of a relative' (HSDU, 1984, p. 21), echoing similar beliefs across the rest of the region.

Patients with an STD are more likely initially to visit the *inyanga* or *sangoma* before seeking help in the formal health care setting, due to the stigma related to STDs (Chapter 3). Stigma is apparent through the scorning attitude of some nurses, and the reluctance to visit the clinic or hospital on the day designated for STD treatment. In Soweto, the reluctance to utilise the formal health sector is also evident, especially for the young: 'they are not using condoms, some fear to ask for them' (female, 15). Similarly in Katutura, Windhoek: 'if you are in school uniform then the nurses will say that children of that and that school, and these small kids are using contraceptives' and 'when you are 14 and you go to the clinic asking for contraceptives they will scold you and ask your parents for permission, but we don't want our parents to know that we are using contraceptives, they are too strict!' (quoted in Hailonga, 1993, p. 18).[19] In fact, the issue of condom use is surprisingly complex, and warrants closer attention.

The Behavioural Politics of Condoms

Condoms are an integral part of STD and HIV/AIDS prevention, and their use has increased significantly over the past decade. Correct use of them reduces the risk of HIV transmission by almost 100 per cent, even though they can still break during use. In sub-Saharan Africa, demand more often than not exceeds supply, as there remain a multitude of problems related to their marketing and distribution. The objections to condoms across Africa however are diverse and manifold, to the extent that even in highly sexually active groups, such as prostitutes, condom use rarely exceeds around 50 per cent, and also varies greatly both within and between high risk groups. In Dar es Salaam, for example, condom use among street children is extremely low (less than 1 per cent), despite the common occurrence of anal intercourse (Iranganyuma, 1993). In Zaire, a study found that condom use between prostitutes and students is unusually low, as the prostitutes consider the students to be more knowledgeable and less liable to be infected (Schoepf, 1993). As mentioned above, evidence from Nigeria suggests that condom use is relatively low in relationships between older men and schoolgirls (Soyinka et al., 1993), and this trend may well be apparent in southern Africa too. The 'sugar daddy' phenomenon has grown in extent partly as a result of the widespread belief that young girls are free of HIV infection, hence the reason for the low incidence of condom use. The 'Anti-AIDS' clubs in Zambian schools sometimes refuse to advocate the use of condoms, as condoms are associated with promiscuity. This association is not without grounding; in Zimbabwe, a study among urban factory workers found a significant association between seroprevalence and condom use (Mbizvo et al., 1993), indicating that those men using condoms are more likely to be involved in high risk relationships. This condom use is evidently inconsistent, and condom use can even be considered as a proxy indicator of high risk sexual activity, rather than vice versa. Regarding adolescents, a sample of Bulawayo students showed a use rate of 9.4 per cent among females, and 16 per cent amongst males (Chisango et al., 1993), while among adults in a separate study only 4.9 per cent of males reported current condom use (Mbizvo and Adamchak, 1989). The accuracy of these surveys must always be questioned considering the inherent problems of surveys of this type and the range of research techniques adopted (Chapter 2). There are also problems related to data such as condom usage rates, as there is often no associated qualitative information regarding the misuse or re-use of condoms, or indeed their 'deliberate' misuse through cutting or perforation, which anecdotal evidence suggests is fairly widespread.

In South Africa, aversion to condom use is the dominant theme, although explanations for this vary; 'cultural beliefs are also a barrier to condom use in South Africa, where many people consider it essential that the sperm of the man actually enters the woman' (Gould, 1993, p. 58). In some townships the lack of electricity, and thus lack of light, makes condom use difficult, as well as the taboo surrounding the exposure (to children) of the genitals, 'so sex takes place in the dark and condoms are generally not accepted' (*AIDS Analysis Africa*, 1993, p. 1). Amongst university students in Cape Town, 13.3 per cent of males and 19.1 per cent of females considered condoms 'against their religion' (Friedland *et al.*, 1991). Of 120 sexually active high school students in Gauteng only 5 reported using condoms on a regular basis (van Aswegen, 1995). Female township school students in Cape Town found problems negotiating their use (Mathews *et al.*, 1990), while all 110 of a sample of urban black mothers questioned in Durban stated that they had never experienced sexual intercourse where their partner had used a condom (Abdool Karim *et al.*, 1991). The highest incidence of condom use was in a sample of goldminers, where 32.6 per cent had used them at least once (IJsselmuiden *et al.*, 1990). In Natal, condom use amongst a sample of Zulu males with GUD was 4 per cent (O'Farrell *et al.*, 1991), and anecdotal reports emphasise the general unpopularity of condoms: 'According to the survey (of Kwazulu schoolchildren aged 17–23, July 1990), a third of respondents believed AIDS to be a "joke" and 90 per cent said that they would never use a condom.'[20]

In my research the issue of condom use in relation to the spread of STDs was mentioned by 8.1 per cent of respondents, with a considerable range of 3 per cent (Lebowa) to 25.2 per cent (Soweto) between the field sites. A clear urban/rural differential has emerged, showing a much greater awareness of condoms in relation to STD prevention in Soweto than in the rural sites. This not only reflects the greater access of condoms in the urban setting, but also the higher exposure of urban communities to education and prevention programmes. The change in awareness about condoms is indeed considerable in the urban setting. In a 1985 study of schoolgirls in a Pretoria township, 91.3 per cent of respondents said that they had never heard of condoms (Du Toit, 1987). Overall, younger rather than older people were more aware of condoms, but this relationship shows no statistical significance. Figure 4.8 shows the clear urban/rural differential in awareness of condoms, with the associated age relationship. Better-off households, overall, are more aware of the lack of contraception, possibly reflecting their higher access to both contraception and information ($p < 0.005$, Figure 4.9). Without multivariate analysis it is impossible to determine whether this outcome is simply the result of the higher average income of the Soweto households, who also have higher access to information. An analysis of the Soweto sample, however, demonstrates the independent influence of income on awareness of condoms.

The contrast between the sites is striking, especially the urban-rural differential in awareness, possibly reflecting the notion in rural areas that condoms are usually perceived to prevent unwanted pregnancy, rather than unwanted infection. The extent of condom use in the different sites is very difficult to quantify

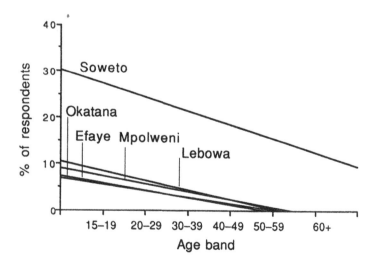

Figure 4.8. Age variable in 'lack of condom use' as a perceived determinant of STD incidence
Note: the lines represented are best fit of the actual data.

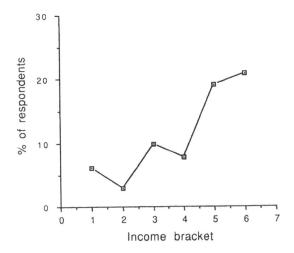

Figure 4.9. Income variable of respondents in 'lack of condom use' as a perceived determinant of STD incidence (all sites) (N.B. most respondents mentioned the lack of condom use in reference to lack of contraceptive use, others mentioned 'contraception' without directly mentioning condoms; see Figure 4.10).

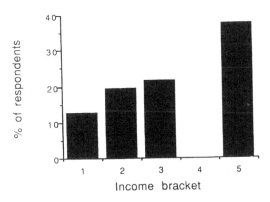

Figure 4.10. Soweto: income as a variable in 'lack of condom use' as a perceived determinant of STD incidence

exactly, but small samples can give indications of the approximate use, or the *perceived* extent of use. In Efaye, respondents who are young and sexually active were asked about condom use and their knowledge of AIDS prevention (Table 4.8).

Table 4.8. Condom use amongst adolescents in Efaye, Natal

Response	Males (%)	Females (%)	Total (%)
Yes	7 (26.9)	2 (4.7)	9 (13.0)
No	19 (73.1)	41 (95.3)	60 (87.0)
Total	26 (100)	43 (100)	69 (100)

Only 13 per cent of respondents claimed they use condoms; a similar figure of 8.7 per cent was obtained from the KAPB survey of school students in Mpolweni. Despite the obvious inaccuracies which are inevitable in a small survey of this type, the differences in male and female responses seem significant. Almost 27 per cent of males claimed that they use condoms as opposed to only 5 per cent of females. Those males who claimed they used condoms did so almost exclusively because of the risk of HIV infection. One respondent even claimed he used condoms but then showed almost complete ignorance regarding HIV transmission. When questioned further on this point he stated that he had heard on the radio that condoms prevented AIDS so he started to use them, but didn't actually know *why*. For the females the reasons given for not using them were related to lack of information on condom use and where to get them. But the gender difference in influencing sexual behaviour was marked. Women could request the use of condoms, but not dictate it within sexual activity, while males would take the decision to use condoms unilaterally, only partly influenced by the wishes of the female. Many girls stated that their boyfriends had either actually refused to use condoms or were likely to refuse if asked. The economic need of girls was posed as a reason why refusal of sex was not an option for many, and this was confirmed by other female respondents. There still remain lingering doubts in the minds of some as to the reality of the AIDS epidemic and one girl in Efaye told me that she would only start using condoms when somebody that she knew developed AIDS.

In Okatana and the Oshakati area, the issue of condoms was

In Okatana and the Oshakati area, the issue of condoms was raised in both the community resident survey and the KAPB survey of students. Their responses are summarised in Table 4.9.

Table 4.9. Condom use amongst adolescents in Oshana

Response	Males		Females		Total	
	Okatana	Students	Okatana	Students	Okatana	Students
	No. %	No. %	No. %	No. %	No. %	No. %
Yes	18 58.1	35 50.7	11 30.6	16 76.2	29 50.9	51 56.7
No	13 41.9	34 49.3	25 69.4	5 23.8	38 49.1	39 43.3
Total	31 100	69 100	36 100	21 100	67 100	90 100

N.B. this table show results from both the Okatana and students surveys. Average age: males 24.0, range = 15–40; females 23.1, range = 15–35.

As in the Natal sample, more males than females in the Okatana sample stated that they are using condoms with their partner, and this of course may be due to varying degrees of honesty amongst the respondents. Amongst the students, however, the reverse is true. Overall, the students claimed slightly higher condom use than the Okatana sample, and this may be due to better access to condoms at the schools as they are mostly located in peri-urban areas.[21] The differences between the female groups is striking, as the female students claimed a much higher condom use than the Okatana females, and even the male students. This may be because of education status, as well as the availability of condoms. The problems of interpreting results from a survey of this type are self evident, but even with these limitations accepted, condom use (and the potential for increased, sustained use) appears to be considerable in the Namibian context, relative to the rural South African sites.

There is an apparent distinction between condoms as contraception and condoms as a means of preventing HIV infection. Medical practitioners in Namibia have noted that condom use is

purposes of contraception (Ahrenson-Pandikow, 1992). A pilot
survey conducted in 1991 (NISER, 1991) indicated that behavioural change was occurring but to a very limited extent, as 75
per cent of respondents indicated awareness of condoms but only
25 per cent claimed to ever use them, with only 7 per cent
claiming consistent condom use. A separate survey claimed that
condom use was as low as 1 per cent (Andima et al., 1994). The
most common contraception prescribed to adolescents is the injected NUR Isterate, followed by the oral pill. Condoms are the
third most prescribed contraception method (NISER, 1991, p.
52). This increased use of condoms is, of course, encouraging,
but anecdotal evidence suggests that their use is very inconsistent, and is mainly determined by their availability. Encouraging
further condom use (and sustaining that use) is a priority, but of
greater importance is increasing the accessibility of condoms.
Many students stated that they would use them if they knew
where to get them. In the more isolated rural areas they are
almost completely unavailable. However, opposition to condoms
is evident in some quarters, not least from the fact that the
hospital in Okatana is Roman Catholic. The official view taken at
the hospital is pragmatic and their use is not actively discour-
aged. At a national scale in both Namibia and South Africa, the
churches have proved to be effective opponents to the advocacy
of condoms but attitudes appear to be changing slowly (Chapter
3). Behavioural response to condoms in the community is generally positive despite the occasional rebuff: 'Some don't want to
use contraception – want flesh to flesh' (male, 29). The principal
problem is really one of accessibility, not acceptance. Nevertheless, problems with acceptance are apparent in certain contexts.
Within marriages or semi-permanent relationships, initiating the
use of condoms may be extremely difficult. Many female respondents stated that if they requested their partner to use a
condom, they would implicitly be accusing the men of infidelity,
or admitting it themselves. This barrier regarding trust prevents
the topic being discussed openly, even though many women tac-
itly accept the likelihood of their (often absent) partners having
other sexual partners. What needs emphasising is this special
vulnerability of married women to HIV infection, and the perva-
sive fatalism which results. The message is that in any one context there are only so many potential condom users; those people
must be reached with information, and the means to access them
must be provided. 100 per cent coverage will never be reached
but every condom used is a success story.

Contextual Control and High Risk Behaviour

The complex milieux of environmental and behavioural influences on sexual activity ultimately manifests itself in individual sexual case histories. Each one will be different, but themes begin to emerge which outline general underlying processes: lack of information, poor access to health care, unequal gender relations, economic pressures and behavioural aspects of sex. With HIV endemic in a community, the reasons for the rapid spread of the virus can be illustrated by some case studies of young people in that community. Asking simple questions to people can reveal these histories – only at a local level can they be properly understood, with possible interventions designed by and for the people in the area. Understanding the situation of people's lives is the first and most crucial step to helping communities construct meaningful prevention schemes. Case histories were gathered in both Mpolweni and Efaye.

Mpolweni

- A 30 year old woman is unemployed and single but has a boyfriend who is a policeman based in Pietermaritzburg. She visits him roughly once a month at his base. She is aware of HIV and its transmission but they do not use condoms, as neither of them want to, even though she has a small stock at home.

- A 19 year old girl is single and unemployed and has a boyfriend who lives in Swayimani. He is 24 and unemployed, and they see each other at weekends. They are not using condoms as she claims that she trusts him. Despite her trust, she considers herself at risk of HIV infection.

- A 17 year old schoolgirl has a boyfriend two years her junior. She has asked him to use condoms but he refuses, and they continue to have a sexual relationship.

- A 23 year old woman is single and unemployed. Her boyfriend is 30 and is a truck driver working within Natal. She sees him at weekends while he is not working. She has asked him to use condoms but he refused; she doesn't know why.

- A 23 year old man is single and unemployed, and claims that he has many girlfriends; 'every day I can get somebody' and points towards the school. He says that he uses condoms which he gets from the clinic in Pietermaritzburg.

- An 18 year old girl is single and unemployed. Her boyfriend is a driver and works in Kwazulu; he comes home once a month. She considers herself at risk of infection but does not want to use condoms.

Efaye

- A 20 year old woman has a boyfriend who is a soldier based in Durban. He visits her twice a year. She is not using contraception but would like more information regarding condoms.

- A 17 year old girl has a boyfriend who works at the nearby Noodsberg Sugar Mill. He stays in the compound at the mill and comes home once a month. She used to use condoms when she lived in Mbali (which has a clinic), but now in Efaye she does not because there is no readily accessible clinic.

- A 21 year old woman, doing Standard 6 at school, has a boyfriend who works in Durban and comes home once a month. He is in his 40s and has many partners in Durban. She wants him to use condoms but he refuses.

- A 32 year old woman is single and unemployed. Her partner is unemployed and living in Johannesburg. He comes home once every three months. She is not using contraception but wants him to use condoms – she has not asked him because she is afraid of him.

- A woman is 21 and doing Standard 7 at school. She is a known prostitute in the village. She says that she has a boyfriend in Durban who is a factory worker, and returns home once a month. She is using DepoProvera but wants to use condoms, however she does not know where to get them. Her father is in Johannesburg while her mother is also a known prostitute.

- A 19 year old girl has a boyfriend working in a garage in Hammersdale, returning home once a month. She is not using condoms but wants to, but states that she has not asked her boyfriend. Even if he refuses she will continue to have sex with him. She then says that he has many other partners.

High risk situations are not necessarily dramatic and easily recognisable; they are not always those involving prostitutes or truck drivers. More often than not they are ordinarily mundane, acted out by people who may not consider themselves at risk of infection. The perception of sexual activity only partly explains the shape of HIV epidemiology. Community recognition of a new, external threat, in the shape of a virus has moulded these attitudes into a form characterised by stigma, fear and fatalism with only limited signs of a positive response. The question to be asked is how are these communities responding to the threat of AIDS, and are these responses going to restrict or encourage the spread of HIV? What are the implications for intervention programmes? These are addressed in the next chapter.

5 Community Responses to HIV/AIDS

Community perceptions of HIV/AIDS take two basic forms: knowledge of the disease, along with methods of transmission and prevention; and the psychosocial construction of the disease, incorporating beliefs relating to its origins and aetiology, risk perception and attitudes towards those infected. The nature of this response to HIV/AIDS is in part conditioned by the macro-determinants of HIV epidemiology (Chapter 3), the behavioural context of sexual activity (Chapter 4) and the heterogeneity within the social make-up of communities, expressed through the responses of individuals. Under examination in this chapter are the perceptions of HIV/AIDS; its representation through fear and stigma in particular, as well as compassionate responses towards those both afflicted and affected.[1] The analysis of the social constructions of the disease is crucial for the formulation of legitimate prevention programmes suited to local conditions, to make them truly *place sensitive* interventions.

Awareness of HIV/AIDS

In the questionnaire surveys, awareness is indicated by the proportion of respondents who mentioned HIV/AIDS when initially questioned 'what is the greatest health problem in the community?'. Respondents could give more than one response, and HIV/AIDS had not been mentioned in the interview prior to the question. The responses given indicate the level of priority accorded to those conditions by the respondent, or, alternatively, due to their topicality within the information networks of the community. Conditions mentioned can be classified as 'AIDS' or 'other', and it appears that conditions mentioned other than AIDS (such as tuberculosis, pneumonia, influenza, gastro-enteritis; Chapter

6) are prioritised wholly through experience of these diseases, whereas HIV/AIDS has a high profile in terms of information and communication networks, which supplements direct experience. For example, a KAPB survey in Ghana revealed that people knew more about AIDS than they did about malaria, despite the far higher death rate for malaria and its long history in the area (Antwi *et al.*, 1993). The subjective environments in which HIV is spreading are more complex than for other diseases, due to the milieu of (mis)information, misconceptions and latent social forces of moral indictment and stigma.

Community 'prioritisation' of HIV/AIDS was highest in Soweto out of the field sites, where 25.2 per cent of respondents mentioned AIDS, and this proved to be the most common response in the Soweto sample. In the rural communities, the proportion mentioning AIDS was much lower, with a range of 2–5.8 per cent (Table 5.1), ranking it well below other diseases such as influenza and tuberculosis (Chapter 6).

Table 5.1. Community prioritisation of AIDS as a health problem

Site	% of respondents mentioning AIDS
Soweto	25.2
Natal 1 (Mpolweni)	5.8
Lebowa	4.0
Oshana (Okatana)	3.0
Natal 2 (Efaye)	2.0

Across the sample as a whole, only several respondents had *not* heard of AIDS when asked (if HIV/AIDS had not been previously mentioned by the respondent), indicating a very high overall awareness of the existence of disease; what varies is the *priority* accorded to the disease. The large disparity between the field sites is likely to be the result of differential exposures to (media) publicity and education programmes, rather than any differences in direct experience of the disease. With HIV prevalence rates being roughly the same in each of the sites (Chapter 1), other factors determining awareness are presumed to be operating, leading to the 'risk environment' as a subjective phenomenon having geographical variation. A crucial aspect of this risk environment is the information available to individuals (X_{1-5}), and this translates as both direct (thick arrow) and indirect linkages (thin arrows), as depicted in Figure 5.1.

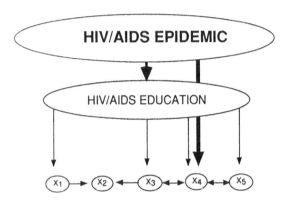

Figure 5.1. Information flow and HIV/AIDS

Information at an individual level has three sources: direct contact with someone who is seropositive or has AIDS, education and prevention initiatives, and inter-personal contacts. In an urban context such as Soweto, the information network is denser, not only in terms of population, but also in terms of the amount of information within the network. For example, a study in Zimbabwe reported that school pupils from homes in urban areas were better informed about AIDS than those from rural areas (Wilson *et al.*, 1989).

Virtually all people have had some information regarding the epidemic, either through direct knowledge concerning people with AIDS (PWA), education programmes, or through inter-personal contacts. Absolute knowledge regarding the disease can be explored by means of KAPB surveys. In the KAPB survey conducted by the author with secondary school students in the Oshakati area of Namibia, for example, all 102 respondents had heard of AIDS, and when questioned, 9 (8.8 per cent) could name only one transmission method correctly, while 48 (47 per cent) and 45 (44 per cent) could name two and three methods respectively. Degrees of knowledge vary according to the actual information sources and the relative impact of the exposures. Someone with high or repeated exposure to education programmes can be considered as a 'net informer' to someone with less exposure. The relative states of inter-personal knowledge are dependent on several factors: the absorption and recall of reliable information, the possible conflicts in credibility between newly received information and pre-existing beliefs/conceptions regarding AIDS and other diseases, and the degree to which information is shared between people, or *who* talks to *whom* about *what*. Education programmes attempt to maximise the information received by individuals regarding the disease, and are now looking to increase the information flow between people by encouraging the discussion of sexuality and sexually transmitted diseases, a theme adopted by the Namibian National AIDS Control Programme. This information flow is often differentiated along the lines of gender, status and age cohort, which has led to the formation of groups with different awareness status. Knowledge levels appear highest in secondary school students, those of higher socioeconomic and educational status and men, while being lowest in 'out of school' youth and women.

From the questionnaire survey, younger people were more likely to mention AIDS as a health problem within the community (Figure 5.2), although the statistical significance of this is

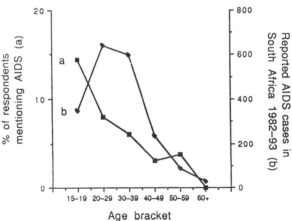

Figure 5.2. Age variation in awareness of AIDS as a community health problem and AIDS deaths in South Africa[2]

not great (p–0.067). It does, however, reflect the partial success of education programmes in raising the awareness of young people, and these programmes must be strengthened, particularly for early-mid teenagers, the 'window of hope generation'. In Zambia, 1994 data from the National AIDS/STD/TB/Leprosy Programme indicate that HIV incidence rates in the 15–19 year age group could well be dropping in urban areas (Fylkesnes et al., 1995), again showing the value and potential success of prevention programmes. The heightened awareness of AIDS amongst teenagers, as a result of education, is also demonstrated by the fact that despite awareness being highest in this younger age group, actual AIDS deaths are most prevalent in the 20–39 age cohorts. The direct correlation between awareness and age cohorts is therefore complicated by both the latency period of the virus and the lack of knowledge of seropositive status for most carriers.

In a situation where the AIDS case rate is very low, visible health problems are the same to most people. There are minor variations, such as diseases or conditions related to old age. During the early stages of the AIDS epidemic, the visual aspects of the disease are very limited, and what is visible may be confused with existing prevalent symptoms or conditions. In Kwazulu, the most common diagnostic criteria for AIDS are currently wasting, tuberculosis, lymphadenopathy (present in 52 per cent of cases) and oral thrush (19 per cent).[3] In the Oshakati/Ondangwa area of Namibia, primary manifestations of AIDS or potential indicators of early HIV infection are tuberculosis, herpes-zoster and wasting.[4] Similarly, tuberculosis, acute pneumonia, herpes-zoster and wasting are the most common presentations of HIV disease and AIDS among adults in Soweto (Karstaedt, 1992). The precise geography of the opportunistic infections may affect the responses to the early stages of the epidemic as the visibility of the disease would depend on the syndromic familiarity of people regarding those with AIDS related complexes (ARCs). HIV infection and AIDS cases are most common in the younger age groups (age 15–35), but there is no relationship between age bracket and 'knowing somebody with HIV/AIDS', so another factor must be determining this relationship. Education programmes targeting the young are thus having some positive effect, as prioritisation appears to be relatively low in the older sexually active age groups, who could be more resilient in relation to behavioural change programmes.

Single people[5] are more aware of AIDS as a community health problem (p<0.05), presumably reflecting their younger and more

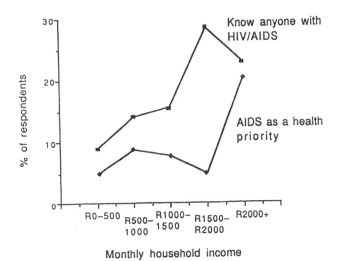

Figure 5.3. Awareness of HIV/AIDS by income group

sexually active profile, and higher likelihood of having many partners. Respondents from better-off households possibly have a higher overall awareness of AIDS as a health problem and are also more likely to know someone with the disease (Figure 5.3; with values of $p<0.01$ and <0.05 respectively). The data show that these relationships are not straightforward, however, indicating the need for some caution in interpretation. Results from a survey in the United States indicate that this process may be universal, as the lowest income groups sampled perceived AIDS to be less serious a problem than the higher income groups (Kronenfeld *et al.*, 1993). This emphasises the subjective nature of the risk environment, and the variability in the prioritisation of HIV/AIDS, which is discussed in detail in Chapter 6.

This association may be due to three factors: a higher access to information regarding the disease, higher access to information regarding community residents, due to both economic and social standing, or that HIV infections and AIDS cases are more prevalent in the higher socioeconomic groups. The latter scenario has certainly been a feature of the early stages of the epidemic in countries in central and East Africa, but this has not been the case in South Africa, where evidence suggests that those from the lowest socioeconomic strata are being most affected by AIDS in these early stages of the (Pattern II) epidemic. The importance of education campaigns is again stressed, but it must be noted that

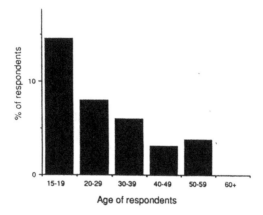

Figure 5.4. Personal knowledge and awareness of people with AIDS amongst respondents, by age group

the difference could be accounted for by the fact that the Soweto sample has a higher economic profile, so implicating the information environment of the urban context *vis-à-vis* the rural. Those with direct experience of the epidemic, through meeting someone who is HIV-positive, or by having personal knowledge of someone who has (died of) AIDS, tend to be in the younger age brackets (Figure 5.4).

The KAPB study of school students in Mpolweni found that 22 per cent knew someone with AIDS, compared to 7.4 per cent in the Mpolweni community sample. This higher awareness reflects both the actual epidemiology of the virus, with its seroprevalence and AIDS case rates, and the targeting of education campaigns, which very often use seropositive persons to talk to school children and youth groups, such as the Township AIDS Project in Soweto. There was considerable variation between the field sites in this aspect of direct contact with the epidemic. Percentages of people who knew of someone with AIDS were as follows: Lebowa 0 per cent, Efaye 4 per cent, Mpolweni 7.4 per cent, Soweto 16.8 per cent and Okatana 27 per cent. Over the whole sample of 528 respondents, 58 (11 per cent) knew of someone with AIDS, while 469 (89 per cent) did not. Some commentators have evidently overestimated the level of direct contact with the disease: 'There are few people left in Africa who do not know someone, or two, or three ... who have died of AIDS' (Gould, 1993, p. 28). In areas of Africa with very high seroprevalence rates, the direct level of personal contact with the disease is proportionately higher. For example, among a sample of students in Uganda in 1992, 75 per cent claimed to have seen someone with AIDS, while 27 per cent had a family member with AIDS, compared to 0 per cent for both categories in 1989 (Bagarukayo *et al.*, 1993). However, a nationwide study of adults in Nigeria found that only 6 per cent knew someone with AIDS (Kigaru *et al.*, 1993), but there the HIV prevalence rate is significantly lower. The variance in direct contact with the disease is striking and shows how the community responses to the disease are based upon differing frames of experience and reference.

This direct contact with the epidemic has the effect of making the epidemic more *immediate*, both temporally and spatially. The epidemic is *here* and *now*. The epidemic has become a component of the 'life worlds' of those people, and the disease is no longer a concern only for *other* people in *other* places. This proximity of the epidemic presumably has important implications for education initiatives, in that positive behavioural responses would be encouraged if it is realised that the disease is, or threatens to be, a local phenomenon. From the survey questionnaires, people who knew of someone with HIV/AIDS were far more likely to mention HIV/AIDS as a community health problem than those who did not (odds ratio 3.5, chi-square $p < 0.001$). This is no surprise, but the important process of *prioritisation* has taken place, and AIDS has taken on more of an immediate profile. This *localisation* of the epidemic has the affect of altering perceptions of the disease, but the changes appear to be only superficial, in that there does not seem to be a fundamental change of attitudes linked to increased awareness. This is discussed in the next section.

Stigma and Sympathy: Community Constructions of HIV/AIDS

Community responses to AIDS can be investigated by examining attitudes towards people with AIDS (PWA). Underlying trends of stigma, fear, ignorance and compassion can be highlighted, and sections of the community with similar perceptions may be seen to form distinct groups. The question was asked, 'what should happen to people with AIDS?'[6] The responses have been classified into three groups: 'kill', 'isolate' (either inside the household, within the community, or external to the community) and 'care'. The category 'care' includes responses related to the proposed treatment of the patient in either the formal or informal health sector. The responses are shown in Tables 5.2 and 5.3.

Table 5.2. Attitudes towards People With AIDS (PWA) (%)

Response	Lebowa	Soweto	Natal 1	Natal 2	Oshana	Ave.
They should be killed	23.0	6.5	22.3	18.0	0.0	14.0
They should be isolated	45.0	55.1	65.3	36.0	74.0	55.1
They should be cared for	9.0	31.8	9.1	62.0	25.0	27.4

Table 5.3. Attitudes towards Relatives With AIDS (RWA) (%)

Response	Lebowa	Soweto	Natal 1	Natal 2	Oshana	Ave.
They should be killed	11.0	6.5	24.0	13.0	0.0	10.9
They should be isolated	57.0	39.3	49.6	21.0	65.0	46.4
They should be cared for	25.0	50.5	22.1	72.0	35.0	40.9

The figures do not always add up to 100, as a small percentage of respondents wanted to isolate the patients while still providing some care function such as food provision, making the categories not mutually exclusive. The figures therefore indicate the number of individuals who mentioned each response independently from other responses. In the minds of the respondents, it was clear that HIV positive status is synonymous with 'having AIDS', and even if the distinction is understood, it is a mere technicality. The tables show that respondents have only marginally more compassion towards family members with AIDS than people with AIDS generally, demonstrating how blurred the distinction can be between individual, household and community. The analysis of community response to HIV/AIDS is essentially an appraisal of the issue of rights; those of the individual *vis-à-vis* those of the community. With AIDS, these interests are often in conflict, and it can be argued that the rights of the individual are, in fact, subordinate to those of the community. This point is not simplistic, however, and generalising across a community is complicated by the polarity of the response.

'They must get what they deserve...'
The desire to see PWA killed is perhaps extreme but has been a universal response to the epidemic. In Britain in the mid 1980s, overt homophobia often culminated in hysterical press reports advocating the killing of PWA and the isolation of homosexuals. In Zimbabwe, in 1994, a member of parliament proclaimed that 'If a pregnant woman is found to have AIDS she should be killed so that AIDS ends with her', moreover, he said, 'the woman would still continue to spread AIDS'.[7] Similarly, in Ghana, respondents in a KAPB survey often advocated 'injectables to kill' for PWA (Antwi *et al.*, 1993). Of a sample of high school students in Gauteng 32 per cent felt that AIDS was a 'punishment for the guilty' (van Aswegen, 1995). There is of course a moral obligation for health workers and community workers generally to vigorously attack such a belief with education. The reasons for these perceptions, however, need to be understood before an appropriate response can be formulated.

The variation between the sites in the proportion wanting PWA to be killed is considerable, ranging from 0 per cent in Okatana to 24 per cent in Mpolweni. The reasons for this variation are not immediately apparent, but certainly the variations in community responses are demonstrated. In Lebowa, 20.2 per cent of respondents said the person should be killed, with the use of an AK-47 being a popular choice. This notion was fuelled by rumours that people found to have AIDS in the Rand townships were being shot (by whom was not clear). A survey of standard 10 pupils in a school in Acornhoek, near to the field site in Lebowa, had revealed similar results. To the question 'what should happen to HIV-positive people?', 27 per cent replied 'they should be isolated', 13 per cent, 'they should be killed'; 12 per cent, 'be hospitalised'.[8] A smaller proportion in Soweto (6.5 per cent) considered killing the best option, and this can be related to the greater destigmatising impact of education programmes in urban areas. The desire to kill was expressed forcefully by some respondents; 'Mercy killing – to prevent spreading, an injection' (female, 29); 'They should be killed because they will infect other people ... or they should be taken to a place where they can stay with people who have the virus ... in the bush' (female, 23); 'they should be killed, because they won't live a long time' (female, 18); 'kill that person ... the person will infect the whole family' (female, 28). One respondent even advocated Nazi methodologies:

> For the survival of mankind such people must be exterminated/killed, for the safety of mankind. Hitler's methods should be applied. There should be compulsory blood tests for everybody. Those testing positive should be killed. (male, 32)

In the Natal communities, high levels of stigmatisation are again apparent; over 70 per cent of respondents would want to see PWA either killed or isolated away from the community. In Efaye, three respondents stated independently that they had heard on the radio that people with AIDS are dangerous and should be killed, so in part determining their response.[9] The particularly hostile reaction of 'kill' may be linked to the violent political climate in the Natal region at the time of the fieldwork, but on further questioning of a group of standard 10 students in Mpolweni, this does not seem to be the case. Violence is an unusually extreme way of resolving conflict or in reaction to a threat, either to the community as a whole (as in the case of AIDS) or in inter-personal disputes. The usual way of resolving conflict situations is said to be through discussion with an attitude of reconciliation. AIDS is perceived to be a unique case in prompting such a hostile response, and is linked mainly to fear which is only partly linked to misconceptions regarding the disease. PWA are perceived to be potential killers rather than ordinary people suffering from a misunderstood illness. In Mpolweni, a higher proportion of respondents stated that they would kill relatives with AIDS than other community members with AIDS. This may be due to the fact that people perceive themselves to be at greater risk of infection if the person lives in the same house, or it could be just ignorant compassion; 'they cannot be helped'.

Sentiments regarding the killing of PWA reflect those of the other sites: 'they must get what they deserve ... shoot them' (female, 33); 'kill them, they can't stay without sex' (male, 23); 'give them [fatal] injection for AIDS' (male, 18); 'kill that person because he might transmit the disease to other people' (female, 27); 'kill all of them' (male, 23); 'shoot them, there is no cure ... you can do nothing for them' (female, 38). In sharp contrast to this severe reaction in the South African sites, in Okatana not one respondent advocated the killing of PWA. Why this response was not offered in Okatana is unclear, but it could be integral to social mores, or possibly relate to the post-war atmosphere which pervades the area. Years of conflict may have left residents with a strong anti-violence ethos. Variety is the theme which must be again emphasised – in making generalisations regarding responses we must be careful of totally misrepresenting the attitudes of large groups of people.

The desire to kill PWA is an extreme response, but is indicative of very high levels of stigma. The extent of the desire to kill is extremely variable, and statistical analysis fails to identify any related factors. For example, an increase in the awareness of AIDS is not supplemented by any marked shift in attitudes, such as changes in the levels of stigma surrounding the disease. Respondents knowing of someone with AIDS are only slightly less likely to consider the killing of PWA as an appropriate response, and are even more partial to the isolation of PWA than those who do not know of someone with AIDS (65.5 per cent as opposed to 54.4 per cent). Both relationships, however, are not statistically significant, but levels of stigmatisation do not seem to be affected by direct contact with the epidemic, and stigmatisation is probably more related to other environmental factors. Indeed, it seems that if a person known to have died of AIDS had had a particularly bad reputation in relation to their sexual behaviour, then stigma and discrimination can be reinforced by the apparent vindication of their death through the disease. For example, in the community of Okatana, one of the local taxi drivers died of the disease. Respondents inferred that he was somehow 'deserving' of his fate. Similarly, in the Lebowan community, rumours suggested that AIDS was associated with local policemen, who had brought it with them from Pietersburg. A popular *shebeen* next to the police station was also associated with the disease, thus implicating both the policemen and the prostitutes who frequent it. In Mpolweni, the disease was commonly associated with prostitutes in Durban and Pietermaritzburg, and with truck drivers, whose main route from the north passes some two kilometres from the village. These localised social identifications of the disease, over and above the grander black, white, or American distinctions, have had the effect of increasing levels of stigma in these early stages of the epidemic. Local myths and stories of the disease may explain what initially seem to be totally irrational responses to the disease.

Stigma and isolation

Stigmatisation is most manifest in the desire to see people with AIDS (PWA) isolated, both socially and geographically removed from the confines of the community. This has been a response common to virtually all areas which have experienced the epidemic to date, and has various historical analogies, particularly in reference to leprosy, syphilis, mental illness and yellow fever. This desire for isolation has certain parallels with the removal and confinement of people who are believed to be witches in parts of the northern Transvaal; a practice which is reputedly on the increase since the election of May 1994. Calls for isolation have been noted across Africa as well as in Western Europe and the United States. The debate regarding the isolation of male homosexuals became a big issue in the United States following the death of the actor Rock Hudson in 1985, and overt homophobia soon took a hold on both sides of the Atlantic. Within Africa, the dissemination of Western press reports could possibly account for the fact that many people believed (falsely) that most PWA in Africa were homosexuals. Homosexuals, though, did not form a group which acted as a social scapegoat to the extent they did in the United States and Europe (except perhaps in South Africa). The stigma was, and is, directed at any groups where infection rates are presumed to be the highest, most noticeably prostitutes (Chapter 4). In a study in Nairobi, 78 per cent of family members and 80 per cent of community members advocated the isolation of patients with AIDS, while the figure was 70–90 per cent for samples of respondents in Ghana (Antwi *et al.*, 1993). A similar survey conducted in Botswana in 1988 found that 75 per cent of respondents thought that PWA should be quarantined (Lesetedi *et al.*, 1989). Stigma is not restricted to adults; an MP in Swaziland said that children with AIDS should be barred from school.[10] In Kenya, President Daniel arap Moi himself had called for the isolation of PWA:

He claimed that there had been an incident where a person had deliberately infected 100 other people. The president said that AIDS patients should be isolated from the rest of society and called on prison officials to see that prisoners with AIDS were identified and isolated from other inmates.[11]

In the field sites, the desire for isolation of PWA was the dominant theme, ranging from 36 per cent in Efaye to 74 per cent in Okatana. In the Soweto sample, over half of the respondents (58 per cent) felt that the PWA should either be isolated in hospital, in a special ward, or in a 'special place' which would prevent them from mixing with the community. These results are consistent with another study of family planning clinic attenders in an inner city clinic in Johannesburg, where 68.2 per cent of respondents felt that AIDS patients should be hospitalised in isolation wards (Govender et al., 1992). While discussing this topic further with respondents, many unwittingly described something very similar to the current Cuban method of isolation as the most desirable response.[12] The emphasis is consistently placed on the notion that the PWA should not be able to mix with uninfected community members: '[They] should be placed in a concentration camp ... be taken good care of ... placed under guard' (male, 26); 'Isolated from healthy people, so build a place for them' (female, 40); 'Isolated in hospital, kept there until they die ... kept away from the community' (female, 23); 'They shouldn't live with normal people, a place should be built for them' (male, 25); 'A place of their own should be built, so that they may get encouragement from other people with the virus ... they'll encourage each other' (female, 35); 'They must be treated like other people; they are also people, but they must live in place of their own, the community should visit them' (female, 21). Many more examples similar to these could be cited.

In the Natal communities of Mpolweni and Efaye, the desire for isolation is again apparent (49.6 per cent and 21.0 per cent respectively). The reasons for the difference between the villages are impossible to define exactly, and are to be found within the social fabric of the communities themselves. Mpolweni, as a mission area, may have moral undertones regarding the attitude towards AIDS, and mild intolerance may be in part due to strong, communal, religious beliefs. In Okatana, levels of stigma are again high, reflecting a trend which is apparent across the whole country, as 69 per cent of respondents felt that PWA should be isolated away from the community, either in a hospi-

tal, or in some sort of camp where they should be confined.
These sentiments of removal and isolation were expressed many
times: 'Isolate in a camp – no contact with others who are not
infected' (male, 50); 'Isolated in a camp so they can make love
with those already infected' (female, 17), and

> They must be caged up to the last day of their life, or they must be
> imprisoned for life in jail. Everybody who is affected must be taken
> to a special place which has cages for AIDS persons. The government
> must take strong measures on behalf of those people who are af-
> fected. (male, 28)

The reasons for wanting isolation are complex but usually relate
to simple fear and resultant stigmatisation. Often transmission
methods are not fully understood, so isolation is perceived to
protect others from passive infection. Some respondents mentioned the fact that those testing positive would want to infect
others, so again protection of the community is the rationale for
the reply. This response has been documented elsewhere, and
PWA are often viewed with suspicion, attributed with either the
incapability of remaining abstinent or the malicious intent of
infecting others.

Having AIDS is associated by some as the result of 'wrong-
doings': 'She/he will be shameful of being living on the earth
[sic]' (male, 21, Okatana). In Okatana, the level of stigma is so
high that some people in the community who have been diagnosed as HIV-positive have hanged themselves due to the fear of
community rejection. I heard of several recent cases of local
hangings while conducting the fieldwork. Some respondents considered the likelihood of 'self kill' so great that isolation would
encourage it: 'the community should look after them, in a camp
they would hang themselves' (female, 41); 'Do not tell them that
they get VIGS [Afrikaans for AIDS] because of self-kill. But you
must tell them to use condoms everywhere' (male, 25). Stigma
also took other forms, such as branding: 'they should be marked
on the arms, so that everyone will know' (female, 32). The level
of stigma is such that the desire for isolation even extends to
family members who have AIDS: 'isolate them within the house,
take care of them, they cannot touch anything in the house'
(female, 21); 'family take care, then take them to the camp when
they become ill' (female, 40); 'we're ready to send him to the
camp or place where AIDS victims are isolated' (female, 24).

The desire for isolation is in conflict with the community

identity with disease in so many African societies. The widespread belief that AIDS has been introduced from the United States may have resulted in the reaction to an 'exotic' disease which is itself extraordinary. The stigma which is so apparent may also be partly a result of its importation, (that is originating in 'the other', however defined), as well as the methods of transmission, which implicates identifiable sub-groups within the community:

> The fear of disease, as the history of quarantine indicates, is not aroused by the simple knowledge of physiological effects of the pathogen, but from an ill-informed consideration of the 'kind of person' liable to become ill, and the habits thought to cause or predispose people to the disease. (Musto, 1988, p. 77)

With AIDS, it can be argued that the response is indeed without precedent. Stigmatisation on this scale is certainly unusual, and must be in some way related to the media hysteria which was aroused in the United States and Europe, from where reports of the disease in part aided the construction of the disease in the minds of many Africans. As Saayman (1991) has noted, 'Isolating a sick person by putting her or him in a hospital where the treatment is fully in the hands of medical experts only, is therefore not only foreign to the African understanding, but basically doomed to failure' (p. 25).

Only in Cuba and Bangladesh has the isolation of PWA been attempted, but the desire for quarantine appears to be universal, at least in the initial stages of the epidemic. Stigmatisation has manifested itself in the African context in a variety of ways. A common occurrence has been the ostracisation of members of AIDS-afflicted families and in Tanzania, Zimbabwe and Uganda, an overall lower level of interaction between school students, and between students and teachers (Kinyanjuni and Katabaro, 1993). In a government report from Zambia (Zambian Ministry of Health, 1993), it is recorded that

> In a recent survey done by Mushinge *et al.* in a study of fishermen and fish traders, it was discovered that AIDS patients were sent out by the leaders of the camp. This was especially so if it was a woman suspected of having AIDS.[13]

Also in Zambia, some seropositive workers have been reportedly committing suicide (Williams, 1990), while in Zimbabwe, there

is much discrimination and ostracism in both village social networks (Mhloyi and Mhloyi, 1990) and workplaces (Williams and
Ray, 1993). One man reported 'coming out' with HIV/AIDS, lost
his job, had been thrown out of his parents home and been
evicted from his lodgings six times, before entering into the care
of a church group.[14] 'In most of the households and villages in
our district', says one counsellor in central Manicaland, 'HIV
infection is the best kept secret' (Saunders, 1991, p. 38).

In South Africa, patterns of stigmatisation have been similar,
with problems specifically associated with relations in the work
place and domestic sphere. Of a sample (size unspecified) of
seropositive women in the Western Cape, only one had told a
family member about her status, fearing ostracism and rejection
(Streble, 1992). In Pietermaritzburg, the experience of counsel-
lors indicates that stigmatisation is so high within the family that
patients request that the family be informed of their HIV status
'only when their health is deteriorating to the extent that they
are on the verge of medical disablement' (Wardell and Radebe,
1994). In Durban, the situation is no different for seropositive
women, as an AIDS counsellor reported:

> 'Their only friends are among each other' she said as she explained
> the harrowing experience young girls have to confront. 'They dare
> not turn to others. They're terrified. They think that here at the
> paediatric clinic there might be spies, pretending to be HIV positive
> mothers in order to gain information on them. It's all so sad.'[15]

In the absence of any leading public figures 'coming out' with
AIDS, the levels of stigma are likely to remain very high despite
the growing AIDS case rate. The need to remain silent regarding
HIV status is the norm for most people in southern Africa, and
the words of Shaun Mellors, an AIDS-activist in Johannesburg,
may only be relevant for a minority of PWA in South Africa who
have access to strong community support services: 'A good friend
of mine, John Pegge, once told me that people with HIV/AIDS
are able to be open about their diagnosis because they have
nothing else to lose. How true that is' (NACOSA, 1992, p. 13).

The distinction between individual and community is all too
apparent in relation to the stigmatisation of AIDS. Above all, the
rights of the community subsume those of the individual; the
suffering of one community member is acceptable if the community is perceived to benefit, or be protected in some way. This
could be a problem for policy makers, who, through international

law codes, are obliged to advocate human rights at the level of the individual rather than the community. In reality, the rights of the individual are mostly negated by perceptions at the community level. The case of Cuba is interesting in this respect, as the isolation of AIDS patients is practised with the apparent condonation of both the patients themselves and the island population as a whole.

Misconceptions regarding transmission still persist, such as the belief that mosquitoes are a vector, and that AIDS has a cure (only 62.6 per cent of the sample of Mpolweni students were sure that there is no available cure), but the desire for isolation is found even in those with a sound knowledge of the disease. The knowledge of HIV transmission, on the whole, is fairly comprehensive among the young people. However, it is not fully comprehended that the concept of 'protection' is something which is a deliberate action, through safer sexual practices or deliberate abstinence, rather than 'protection' through the isolation of those infected. The 'protection' is not simply from the virus, it is from some sort of moral contamination, which is itself poorly understood, and wholly associated with 'the other', both racial and social:

> As sickness in Africa is thus understood completely in terms of the community, it is not strictly speaking an individual who falls sick: the sickness of a single member of the community affects the life force of the total community. In the same way, it is not a disease that has to be healed, but a community. (Saayman, 1991, p. 25)

Moreover, the politicisation of the disease in South Africa has created a situation where those infected are somehow affected by a disease which is perceived to be 'artificial', contrary to conditions which are both familiar and more 'natural'. Of the sample of Mpolweni students, 27 (60 per cent) agreed with the statement 'AIDS is a virus invented to control the population'.

The responses listed in Table 5.4 from the KAPB survey of Mpolweni secondary school students, indicate the persisting unclarity surrounding the disease in terms of its aetiology, the 'correct' moral position in relation to AIDS, and the various manifestations of the stigmas concerning the disease. Overall, the high levels of stigma may be a factor inhibiting behavioural change: by wearing a condom, for example, a person would be seen as acknowledging some sort of linkages with a sub-group (such as those who are HIV-positive), a group which is ostracised

Table 5.4. Perceptions of AIDS amongst secondary school students, Mpolweni Mission, Natal (%)

Statement	Yes	No	Not sure
'AIDS is God's way of punishing people who are immoral'	31.8	20.5	47.7
'AIDS is God's way of controlling the population'	13.6	43.2	43.2
'AIDS is a punishment for immoral activities'	38.6	29.5	31.8
'Only disgusting people get AIDS'	11.4	55.8	31.8
'Whites are responsible for spreading AIDS'	18.2	25.0	56.8
'No-one is to blame for AIDS'	33.3	20.0	46.7
'PWA get what they deserve'	56.8	13.6	29.5
'Groups to support PWA are a good thing'	61.4	9.1	29.5
'People who have tested positive for AIDS should not be allowed to have sex'	53.5	16.3	30.2
'PWA should be isolated from other people'	22.7	59.1	15.9
'PWA should be marked so everyone can see them'	52.3	20.5	27.3
'PWA should be avoided as far as possible'	72.7	11.4	15.9
'PWA should stop having sex altogether'	71.1	8.9	20.0
'AIDS patients should be confined together away from society to protect people who are not infected'	59.1	22.7	18.2
'Names of AIDS patients should be published so everyone can know who is infected'	40.0	42.2	17.8

Table 5.4 *continued*

Statement	Yes	No	Not sure
'Those who we know are carrying the AIDS virus should be killed so they cannot spread this terrible virus'	8.9	57.8	33.3

N.B. In the questionnaire the statements do not appear in the order listed above. They have been grouped here by subject, to aid analysis. Multiple answers were permitted, so the percentages refer only to the proportion of students citing a particular perception.

and feared by the community. People wanting to remove themselves from this acknowledged association, may deliberately *not* change their behaviour, in order to emphasise to others their lack of vulnerability and freedom from suspicion. They then, of course, become more vulnerable to infection as prevalence rates in the community rise.

Variance within community stigmatisation
Evidence from the field sites suggests that stigma regarding HIV/AIDS is differentiated along gender lines. Females were more likely to respond 'kill' in response to PWA than males (p=0.053), confirming other reports that women fear the threat of AIDS more than men. A study in Nigeria (Kigaru *et al.*, 1993), found that women, overall, were less knowledgeable about AIDS and considered it a more serious threat than men. This difference has also been noted in the United States (Kronenfeld *et al.*, 1993), and possibly relates to both the lack of knowledge of the disease and/or the universal issue of the relative lack of power for women in negotiating sexual behaviour.

Across the field sites, it is also apparent that the desire to isolate PWA is highest in the poorer households (Figure 5.5), possibly indicating the lack of resources for caring in these households, combined with poorer access to information regarding the disease. A separate national study amongst parents found similar results: 27 per cent of a literate sample felt that PWA should be isolated compared to 70 per cent of a corresponding illiterate group (Conradie and Rabie, 1993).

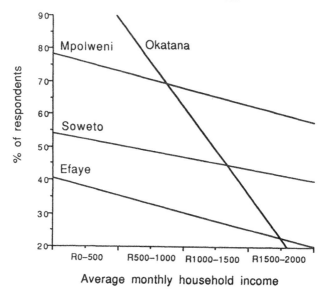

Figure 5.5. Desire to see PWA isolated, by income bracket and area

N.B. The Lebowan field site is excluded as data on income were not collected. The graph shows best fit correlations.

In Côte d'Ivoire, a study of PWA (Mattossovich *et al.*, 1993) revealed that 26.3 per cent of the lowest socioeconomic status group in the sample had been rejected, blamed or isolated by their family, compared to 6.1 per cent of the 'low' class and none from the higher classes (p<0.005). Stigmatisation is thus concentrated in the lowest socioeconomic groups. Univariate analysis failed to reveal any further associations relating stigma to various socioeconomic factors (for example age, household dependency ratio, awareness of AIDS). The relationship between education, poverty and stigmatisation are clear, and points to the need for separate targeting of different socioeconomic groups.

The compassionate response
Across the sample of 528, 27.3 per cent of respondents replied that people with AIDS and 40.9 per cent for relatives with AIDS should be cared for in some respect, either by the community as a whole or by family members themselves. A caring response is also indicated by answers involving taking the patient to traditional healers for treatment, but this forms only a small propor-

tion of this response (less than 5 per cent). Again there is wide variation between the field sites, with a range of 9 per cent (Lebowa) to 62.0 per cent (Efaye) for the caring response to PWA, and 22.1 per cent (Mpolweni) to 72.0 per cent (Efaye) for the caring response to a relative with AIDS (RWA). The village with the lowest number of respondents expressing compassion was Mpolweni Mission, where the KAPB survey amongst secondary school students revealed an ambivalent attitude towards PWA (Table 5.5).

Table 5.5 Attitudes towards PWA amongst secondary school students, Mpolweni Mission, Natal (%)

Statement	Yes	No	Not sure
'I would spend some time with a PWA'	18.2	52.3	29.5
'I would not mind living in the same house as a PWA'	45.5	31.8	22.7
'I would not mind working with a PWA'	54.5	15.9	29.5
'I would not mind looking after a PWA'	25.0	36.4	38.6

In the Soweto community sample, which is relatively compassionate compared to the rural field sites (higher levels of sympathy have also been recorded in urban rather than rural Uganda; Konde-Lulu et al., 1993) sympathy was often mixed with the advocacy of rather Draconian social measures involving the restriction of movement and sanctions on sexual behaviour: 'need to be loved, treated as normal humans – not outcasted' (male, 28); 'be friendly with them ... give support ... special place to keep them' (female, 17); 'they should live with the community, but they shouldn't have sex' (male, 16). For relatives with AIDS, the sentiments are similar: 'encourage him not to be involved in a sexual relationship. He or she should stay at home' (female, 29); 'if the patient wants to announce it [HIV status], then send to a special place – if not, then encourage him to use condoms and care for him' (male, 23); 'encourage him, if he works he can continue until he is no longer able' (male, 16); 'support them and live with them, keep them company, so that they don't feel lonely' (female, 18); 'spread the word that the person has AIDS so that people can be aware. The person can stay with the family' (male, 18); 'seek information on how to treat a person who is infected, he/she will stay with the family but he/she will do everything separately, for example washing' (male, 17).

Community response to relatives with AIDS is, as expected, more compassionate than to PWA generally, and 40.9 per cent of respondents would take care of a relative who is HIV-positive. This indicates a situation where psychological support will come primarily from the family in contrast to a possibly more hostile community. All this, of course, depends on the actual knowledge of HIV status and families inevitably want to protect infected members from ostracism by keeping HIV status, if it is even known, a closely guarded secret.

In Natal, there is a marked difference in some of the responses between the two communities. It is apparent that the Efaye community has a far less hostile reaction than Mpolweni towards PWA; there is stigma in both communities, but far less so in Efaye. Efaye is reputed to be a very close knit community with strong social networks. These networks defy poverty (Efaye has half the average income of Mpolweni), and possibly the common problem of poverty strengthens the community spirit. In Mpolweni, which is economically far more stratified, social linkages are possibly weakened as people become less reliant on each other. Mutual interdependence in Efaye is a communal response to a dominant problem: that of poverty, and communal caring for PWA maybe a simple concomitant of this ethos. This is contradicted, however, by the evidence cited above, that PWA in the lowest socioeconomic households actually experience the greatest amount of stigma. The point is obviously not a simple one, and may implicate factors other than socioeconomic status *per se*, such as the levels of economic stratification and/or strengths of reciprocity networks within communities, as well as religious beliefs.

The compassion which is found in the two Natal villages is again a mixture of altruism and social sanction in relation to relatives with AIDS: 'stay with them ... maybe the whites will help' (female, 17); 'they must stay in the house in a bedroom' (male, 19); 'won't allow him to drink alcohol – it will weaken him, and avoid him if he gets cut' (female, 43); 'the family will look after, but [we] don't like them' (male, 25); 'take them to the doctor and he should decide what to do' (male, 24).

In Okatana, the compassionate response is also evident, but to a lesser extent. For PWA and relatives with AIDS, 25 per cent and 34 per cent of respondents respectively stated that either the community or the family should take care of them. The government was seen to play a minimal role in welfare provision. In reality, the extended family will be the main welfare providers and any community response to this effect should be encouraged: 'the family should look after, and the hospital should supply condoms' (female, 31); 'keep it as a secret and treat them as a human being' (male, 27); 'those who get AIDS, they are not criminals. The better way is just to leave them' (male, 24); 'they must be taken care of and the community must try by all means not to disappoint them or deceive them or separate them from the others' (male, 29).

Across the whole sample, females were more likely to state that a family member with AIDS should be cared for (p<0.005), indicating the more compassionate, 'maternal' role of the women in the household. This attitude does not extend beyond the household to external community members with AIDS, indicating the extent to which the family unit (both nuclear and extended) is the scale of greatest reciprocal obligation and at which initial coping is expected to occur. In Zambia, studies of coping strategies in AIDS affected households indicate that the extended family is receiving minimal support from either the community, NGOs or the government. In one study in Ndola only 15 per cent of the families had received any extra-familial support of any type (Rossi and Reijer, 1995).

Community Responses to AIDS Orphans: Whose Responsibility?

Much concern has been raised over the growing number of AIDS orphans in southern Africa, with an estimated 500,000 expected in South Africa alone by the turn of the century. Research in central and East Africa has shown that this group has had to face many problems relating to social marginalisation and economic survival. The growing number of street children in urban Kenya, for example, can be attributed to the increase in AIDS orphans, who are forced to move, due to either ostracisation and/or the lack of community support in their home areas.

Understanding community perceptions and expectations regarding the welfare of these children is crucial if appropriate community coping mechanisms are to be formulated at an institutional level. The respondents were asked 'what should happen to the AIDS orphans?' Responses have been classified into just two categories to aid analysis. The results are summarised in Figure 5.6.

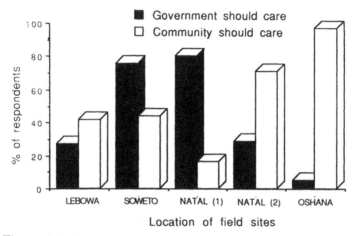

Figure 5.6. Community responses to AIDS orphans in South Africa and Namibia

N.B. Totals do not equal 100, as several respondents mentioned both government and community care, while a considerable proportion of respondents in the Lebowan sample 'did not know'. N = 529.

Overall, the communities are fairly divided as to where the responsibility for the welfare of the orphans lies, with a small majority (52.5 per cent) in favour of community provision, in the households of either relatives or other community members. The desire to see the government care for the orphans averages 45.3 per cent, but varies widely across the sites, with a range from 5 per cent (Oshana) to 80.2 per cent (Mpolweni). The reverse pattern is seen for those wishing to see the community care for the orphans, with a low of 16.5 per cent in (Mpolweni) and high of 97 per cent in Okatana. With responses to orphans in Soweto (the only urban sample), the community actually disclaims most of the responsibility, as 75.7 per cent state that the government should provide for them in some way, mainly through the provision of orphanages. This may reflect the tacit acknowledgement of the lack of community resources which could be used for coping, or simply reflect a high level of stigma attributed to the orphans, as well as their deceased parents. Encouraging, though, is the fact that 43.9 per cent of respondents would want to see the orphans cared for by family members or within the community itself. Some respondents obviously feel that both the government and the community have a caring role to play. What compassion that is apparent must be strengthened to ensure that the orphans do not become a 'parasitic' and an unwanted community within a community: 'orphanage; relatives should not be involved, because as these children are growing, they [the relatives] wouldn't understand them' (female, 26); 'government should take care – a home should be built especially for such kids. Relatives can contribute if they so wish' (male, 46); 'Orphanage; it is not good for the relatives to take them, they sometimes abuse them' (male, 22); 'welfare, government ... relatives are suspicious' (female, 16). In the Natal communities, this division is again apparent between internal and external care; 'there is no-one to look after them, the relatives will take no responsibility ... [they will] become street children in the city' (male, 53); 'the community should look after the children' (male, 25).

Variations in the response to AIDS orphans across the field sites hide trends which are common to all the sites. There are two scales of social construction occurring: that of the 'community ethos' and, at a smaller scale, the definition of sub-groups within the communities, which show similar response profiles regardless of the overall community attitude. For example, people knowing (of) someone with AIDS generally display more sympathy regarding the AIDS orphans. This was apparent through an increased preference for the orphans to be cared for within the community, rather than through governmental orphanages ($p < 0.05$). This emphasises the importance of using people with AIDS in AIDS education programmes in relation to destigmatising those directly affected by the epidemic. With respect to age differentials, an interesting finding emerged in that those who are themselves likely to be dependants – teenagers and those in old age – were least likely to take a sympathetic approach to the orphans, instead emphasising the role of the government in their care (Figure 5.7 overleaf).

Those of parental (and child producing) age were the most likely to want to see the orphans cared for within the community, either within the family unit, or at an inter-household level. Dependants are possibly aware of the limitations of the house-

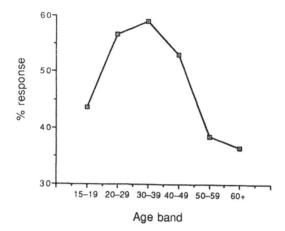

Figure 5.7. 'Community care' for AIDS orphans: response by age group (all sites)

hold budget and realise their vulnerability in a situation where further strain is placed on the household resource base. Differences in opinion are also apparent when considering household income, and it appears that three groups can be identified in terms of economic status: lower, middle and upper income groups. A more sympathetic response is apparent in the extremes

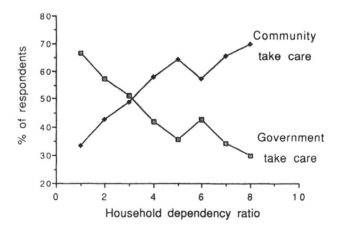

Figure 5.8. Attitudes towards AIDS orphans by household dependency ratio

of the economic spectrum, the poorest and the most affluent households. The sympathy from the poor households could be a function of the 'culture of poverty' and the high awareness of *need* within the community, and the overall familiarity with coping in the face of socioeconomic adversity. This process has been observed in Kagera, Tanzania, where households experiencing adult deaths from AIDS have been more likely to take on foster children from other households. Whether this is because of compassion or the need for extra household labour is unclear. This welfare provision response is virtually absent in the middle-economic group surveyed, who see the government as the primary care givers and claim little responsibility themselves. Amongst the wealthiest households, economic pressures are not so great, and the perceived burden of extra household members is possibly more acceptable, given the assumed flexibility of the household budget. In relation to this aspect of household dependency ratio (ratio of dependants to income earners), results indicate that households with high ratios are more sympathetic towards the orphans. Again, the high awareness of the need of those most economically marginalised could explain this compassionate attitude, which is much rarer in households with low dependency ratios (Figure 5.8).

Research in Kagera, Tanzania, has shown that the dependency ratio is higher in households where an adult has died compared to where death has not occurred. The number of children per adult is 0.94 in AIDS afflicted households, compared to 0.88 for those unaffected (World Bank, 1993). As a result, AIDS has the effect of compounding poverty in households by increasing the dependency ratios. However, the highest levels of compassion, paradoxically, are being displayed in households where the resources are already being stretched by high ratios. It appears that those least able to offer assistance are those who are most willing to provide it.

What appropriate institutional response?

The importance of analysing the perceptions relating to the future welfare of AIDS orphans is that a negative response within communities cannot feasibly be accommodated by institutional bodies. The likelihood is that the number of street children will rise, creating a small but growing sub-culture amongst the youth prone to crime (which is already a serious problem), prostitution and drug abuse (Webb, 1996b; Richter, 1995). Ostracisation of the orphans could lead the children and adolescents into a deprivation cycle, which in the long term could increase their chances of HIV infection, as research in Uganda has indicated. Bagarukayo *et al.*, (1993) reported that a girl from a family with AIDS had a relative risk of 2.32 of being sexually active as compared to a girl who had no family member with AIDS (significant at 95 per cent). No explanation was given for this finding but it is arguably the result of increased social neglect and economic stress. Community tolerance of street children within this deprivation cycle would inevitably be short-lived or non-existent, as the government is seen to be the main welfare provider for these children amongst the urban sample. Orphanages have had limited success in the central African context, such as in Uganda, where they have proved to have been impossible to capitalise and operate, while they also promoted the breakdown of the traditional system of fostering. Orphanages have many sociological drawbacks: neglect, underfunding which can cause malnutrition, lack of adequate socialisation, and the possible lack of education. They are unlikely to be instituted in the southern African context on a wide scale due to this myriad of problems, not least those financial, and NGO efforts in Soweto, for example, are in keeping the children in AIDS afflicted families fed and in school, while empowering them for economic independence following the deaths of their parents. Reciprocity networks within the communities will be tested in relation to the orphans, and the possible failure of family networks, combined with the failure of community networks will result in growing numbers of street children, which can only have a destabilising effect on community structures. Reciprocity within social networks must be identified and somehow strengthened institutionally, such as through youth support groups, vocational training for young people and the training of community outreach workers to monitor the welfare of orphans and orphan households. In addition, education programmes must emphasise that the welfare provision for orphans is primarily the responsibility of the relatives and that institutional response can only supplement, rather than replace community support systems.

The perceptions regarding AIDS orphans show that there are significant levels of compassion which can be investigated and built upon through the institutionalisation of community support systems. The widespread expectation that the government can cope adequately with the impending orphan crisis, however, is a cause for concern, and the lessons learnt in central Africa should not be ignored in the South African context. Caution should be used throughout the planning process, and sensitivity to local conditions, through the recognition of the geography and inherent variability of the social constructions of the disease, is vital if mitigation and coping initiatives are to be appropriate. Indeed, South Africa has much to learn from the experiences of Zambia in relation to orphans and AIDS affected households.

Orphans in Zambia: the limits of family coping
AIDS mortality rates in Zambia are still rising (Chapter 1) and as a result the number of orphans will continue to rise well into the next decade, only stabilising around six years after national HIV prevalence rates have peaked. The spatial variability of the epidemic means that orphan numbers are highest and most concentrated in the urban and peri-urban centres. A 1993 national survey found that 42 per cent of urban households contained an orphan compared to 33 per cent in rural ones (Mulenga, 1993). The National AIDS/STD/TB/Leprosy Programme in the Ministry of Health puts the number of orphans at around 200,000–250,000 in 1995, increasing to 550,000–600,000 by the year 2000 (Fylkesnes *et al.*, 1995).

As far as status of orphans is concerned, several enumeration studies have been completed (Table 5.6 overleaf) The sample sizes vary as do the definitional criteria, but a consistent picture is emerging. The trend is one of a predominance of paternal orphans (those who have lost their father), but the reasons for this are not entirely clear. As far as AIDS related mortality is concerned, it could indicate that either the man is being infected before his partner (and most likely infecting her) or that men progress to AIDS from HIV infection quicker than females. Over time the ratio of paternal, maternal and double orphans will change as the proportion of double orphans increases. The ratio is currently 2.3:0.7:1 and will stabilise when the mortality rate peaks, which is estimated to be well into the next decade.

The issue of paternal, maternal and double orphan status is important in that the average conditions of the different orphans will vary. Double orphans are potentially in the most vulnerable situation and currently rely heavily on the extended family. The difference in welfare status between the paternal and maternal orphans is difficult to clarify without in-depth research. What is certain is that widowers are tending to remarry soon after the death of their wife, whereas widows find it very difficult to remarry. The enumeration survey in Libala and Chilenje compounds in Lusaka of 95 families containing 300 orphans[16] found

Table 5.6. Orphan enumeration studies conducted in Zambia

Location	Year	Paternal (%)	Maternal (%)	Double (%)	Non-enrolment rate (%)
Matero (Lusaka)[a]	1991	61.0	25.0	14.0	32(urban)
National[b]	1993	52.1	24.2	23.7	32 (urban) 68 (rural)
Katete[c]	1993	42.0	27.7	31.0	61 (rural)
Masvingo (Zimbabwe)[d]	1994	75.0	20.7	4.3	NA
Chikankata[e]	1995	45.1	4.7	50.3	53 (rural)
Libala (Lusaka)[f]	1995	65.0	7.4	27.4	NA
Monze[g]	1995	NA	NA	27.8	67.3 (rural)
Ndola[h]	1995	58.6	18.8	22.4	46.4 (urban)
Average		57.0	18.4	25.1	36.8 (urban) 62.3 (rural)

Sources: a Children in Distress Project (1991); b Mulenga, C. (1993);
c St. Francis' Hospital, Katete (1993); d UNICEF/Zimbabwe (1994);
e Chikankata Hospital data (1995), unpublished; f Regiment Parish
(Libala, Lusaka) records (1995), unpublished; g Data from District
Social Welfare Office, Monze, (1995) unpublished;
h Rossi and Reijer, (1995). NA = Not Available

that nearly half of the carers of the orphans are the mothers, a
figure similar to that in Katete (45 per cent). Surviving fathers,
unlike surviving mothers, are unlikely to be care givers (6.3 per
cent) and maternal orphans, who make up 18.4 per cent of the

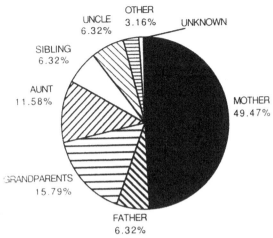

Figure 5.9. Breakdown of carers of orphans in AIDS affected households, Libala Compound, Lusaka

total, are more often than not cared for by other relatives. In none of the cases are the carers outside of the extended families. In 6 per cent of orphan households elder siblings (who are technically orphans themselves) are caring for the orphans, and in all of these cases the siblings were over 18 and usually providing some household income. A breakdown of the carers is provided in Figure 5.9.

Needs assessments of these children indicate that food security, health, education and protection are the major issues at a material level. For example, with educational status, in urban areas estimates put the proportion of orphans of school going age who are not enrolled at 32 per cent, compared to around 25 per cent of non-orphans. In rural areas the situation is more severe, with 68 per cent of orphans not enrolled, compared to 48 per cent of non-orphans. Hospital initiated home based care programmes have generally failed to go beyond the medical attention of the patient to look at the needs of the affected children. The dependency switch in the household as parents fall ill is offset to some extent by help from other family members, but the impact of this reverse in the dependency relationship will become more severe over time as family support is stretched further. Anecdotal evidence suggests that extended families at this stage are still managing to cope with the burden of orphans, with the caring function remaining with the mothers and maternal relatives. In urban settings the coping strategies of the AIDS affected households are mainly informal sector marketeering. Commonly the mother or aunt will sell salaula, charcoal, cooking oil, kapenta, buns, eggs, rice, fritters, vegetables or bread. The profit margin from these activities is very low; as low as ZK1,500 per week in one case (about £0.75). Other income comes from sub-letting. In rural areas coping strategies are far more related to farming activities and brewing beer, with marketeering (buying and reselling) of less importance.

Intra-community support appears to be extremely limited and what help there is comes from institutions such as the churches, the Public Welfare Assistance Scheme within the government, small NGOs and some home based care programmes. Even so, a Ndola survey of orphan households revealed that in 86.4 per cent of cases there was no support from the community, NGOs or the government (Rossi and Reijer, 1995). NGOs have attempted to provide support to orphans and widows through various means such as the Kwasha Mukwenu project in Lusaka, where women 'caretakers' visit and monitor the progress of orphans in their catchment area of households. Other programmes such as drop-in centres are involved in food provision, education and recreation but they are all very small scale and under-funded.

Extended families are still managing to cope and support programmes must aim to target the family as the 'coping unit'. Larger programmes must find ways of supporting this unit. Assistance can take the form of small income generation schemes for widows and vocational training for orphans, in both small scale manufacturing and service activities. At the community scale small agricultural schemes are being managed with the profits going to those most in need as decided by the project committee. Pilot projects are underway across Zambia, but questions still remain regarding the management capacity of communities in relation to these projects, the feasibility of income generation schemes in a severe economic environment, and how the ownership of community projects can be transferred from institutions such as churches and hospitals to self administering community structures. It is a time of experimentation as regards these projects, and there will be failures, but by building on existing coping mechanisms with rotating credit and small technical inputs for example, strong aspects of sustainability can be introduced. The scale of the problem is so large that interventions must be low cost and community centred, and combined with awareness raising of community leaders as to the nature of the orphan problem and the potential solutions.

The overall ambivalence of the responses towards AIDS and those it affects encountered in the field sites must be addressed in education programmes. Ignorance regarding methods of transmission is a contributory factor towards high levels of stigma and the provision of technical information must not be neglected within the programmes, despite evidence of an overall high awareness of the disease. The stigmatisation of the disease will undoubtedly continue in the short term, but it can be removed through the acknowledgement by public figures who have the disease, combined with the increased use of PWA in education programmes. Stigma which remains at high levels is a serious impediment to prevention initiatives, as discussion regarding sexual behaviour is restricted. The perceptions of AIDS reviewed above show that there are significant levels of compassion which can be investigated and built upon through the institutionalisation of community support systems. But caution should be used, and sensitivity to local conditions, through the recognition of the geography and inherent variability of the social constructions of the disease, is vital if prevention initiatives are to be appropriate. This approach to HIV/AIDS prevention is only part of the solution as attitudinal change all too often occurs when the epidemic has already taken a hold within a community. The next chapter addresses this problem in the light of what development processes can contribute to HIV/AIDS prevention and argues for the realisation of an holistic approach within prevention planning.

6 The Development of HIV/AIDS Prevention Programmes

The complexity of both the socioeconomic context of the epidemic and the responses which it has generated underlines the need for a prevention package which itself is wide ranging and holistic in its conception. For an HIV/AIDS prevention package to be effective, issues within the environment which affect sexual behaviour have to be addressed, as well as the behavioural motivations of individuals. The preceding chapters have shown the importance of this dual concept, but the translation of these notions into a workable policy is extremely problematic, as different time perspectives need to be integrated into the same programme. The identification of factors within the socioeconomic environment, which are partly determining the shape of the epidemic, is a useful and necessary exercise, but unless this identification can provide policy guidance, the exercise remains academic. The attribution of causation to macro-structures operating within any context in relation to HIV epidemiology is a sure way to incite frustration and possibly fatalism in the minds of those attempting to halt the spread of HIV and of people vulnerable to infection generally. Pointing fingers at social processes such as migrant labour and 'poverty', as well as natural phenomena such as drought, can lead to an ethos of hopelessness. This must be avoided at a local scale as far as health workers and NGOs are concerned, as these macro-processes are beyond the scope of any intervention programme. However, the recognition of the crucial role of certain structures and contexts remains, leading to suggestions that NGO efforts in prevention are mostly futile, in that the scope of their interventions can be no more than in building infrastructure, leaving the wider societal problems unchanged, due to the lack of political will for their transformation. The resultant theme of programmes has necessarily been on curing symptoms rather than addressing causes, but too little practical attention has been placed on contextual factors which *can* be mitigated at a local scale. This poor conceptualisation of HIV/AIDS prevention in the past, through the creation of the myth that AIDS is a medical issue requiring solely or primarily medical intervention, has resulted in programmes which were destined to fail.

The Failure of Short Term Interventions

There is no doubt that, in sub-Saharan Africa, AIDS prevention efforts have met with extremely limited success. The increasing HIV rates across the region are testament to this simple conclusion (Chapter 1). Explanations for this widespread failure have been offered but a programmatic shift is still lacking. The few recorded successes have been in geographically specific core target groups, through initiatives in the private sector, most notably amongst prostitutes, truck drivers and mine and plantation workers. For example, Williams and Ray (1993) describe how there has been a considerable decline in the number of reported STDs at workplaces in Zimbabwe due to schemes at mines and commercial estates, where drops of 53 per cent to 75 per cent have been reported. In the Eastern Highlands Tea Estates from 1991–93 there was a drop of 59 per cent. Chipfakacha (1993) described a programme with prostitutes at a mine compound in Shurugwi in the Midlands Province of Zimbabwe, which reported a 74 per cent drop in the number of STD cases. These intensive programmes involved the targeting and treatment of STDs with patient–partner follow up, condom provision, and closely monitored peer education initiatives.

The evaluation of such schemes is essential, and 'success' is quantified through the measurement of condom usage rates and STD prevalence/incidence rates in the population under surveillance. The impacts of these programmes, however, have been socially and geographically limited, with the course of the wider epidemic unchanged. While recognising that conventional indicators may not be sensitive enough to pick up any changes which have occurred in the general population, Lamptey *et al.* (1993) suggest that large scale national programmes have not had an impact because of three factors:

• Interventions have been localised, with limited socio-geographic impact.

- There has been a lack of comprehensiveness within prevention programmes. The three themes within prevention: reduction of high risk behaviour, provision of condoms and the reduction in prevalence of STDs, are only very rarely integrated in a single intervention. STD programmes have proved to be the weakest in their extent, mainly due to financial restrictions.

- There has been a lack of supportive policies such as education in schools, appropriate church support and condom advertising.

These explanations are only part of the reason for the widespread failure of AIDS prevention programmes, which are typically characterised by short term, technical interventions, concentrating on the prevention of the actual transmission of the virus. This approach has failed to address the actual socioeconomic *context* of sexual behaviour as well as the issues surrounding the social relevance of education programmes and community constructions of the disease (Chapter 5), which themselves have a direct effect on the levels of HIV transmission in any one locality. Paradoxically, the conceptual models of the epidemic have increasingly stressed the structural aspects at the expense of the role of agency, whereas prevention programmes have failed to grasp the significance of these developments. The gradual realisation, for example, that education is only a contributory factor in causing behavioural change, rather than its prime mover, has taken too long. As Schoub (1992, p. 55) commented:

> Education on its own ... is insufficient to effect sustained behavioural changes in the population, and the well-worn aphorism 'education is the only vaccine' is simplistic and naïve.

Education is only one of three major determinants of behavioural change. Agents must also want to change their behaviour and have the behavioural/social skills necessary to execute such a change. The Information, Motivation and Behavioural Skills Model expounded by Fisher and Fisher (1992) goes some way to conceptualising the psychological processes involved (Figure 6.1).

An individual must know about the disease, want to change his or her behaviour, and be in a position that allows for behavioural change. These factors themselves have varying determinants, making the knowledge–behaviour change link very

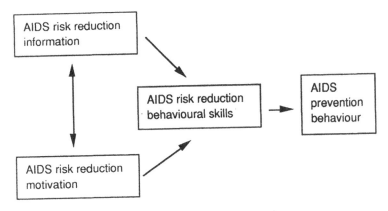

Figure 6.1. The Information, Motivation and Behavioural Skills Model, after Fisher and Fisher, 1992

inconsistent and socio-geographically specific. Short term interventions in sub-Saharan Africa have made significant impact only in one of the three areas, that of AIDS risk reduction information. As has been shown in Chapter 5, levels of awareness of AIDS are very high in southern Africa, yet the links with attitudinal and behavioural changes are very tenuous. Levels of stigmatisation, for example, are not significantly diminished through personal knowledge of someone with the disease, although this knowledge may have direct impact on levels of behavioural change. The links between personal knowledge, stigma and behavioural change need to be researched further, as they have direct implications for *inter alia* prevention programmes using peers and PWA as educators. Moreover, in order for the prevention efforts to be effective, the remaining two areas, motivation and behavioural skills, need to be understood and accounted for. Motivation, firstly, is a function of both information and the level of priority accorded to the disease; in other words, the levels of perceived *vulnerability*.

Risk and vulnerability
The subjectivity of the concept of 'risk' has been demonstrated in relation to the perception and behavioural response to a whole variety of environmental risks, both natural and technological. The social constructions of AIDS described in Chapter 5 are integrally linked to attitudes regarding the perceived vulnerabil-

ity of individuals to infection. This, in turn, relates to behavioural responses and the whole milieu of contextual and psychological determinants of those responses. For example, Linden *et al.* (1991, p. 993) reported from a study in Rwanda:

> Women who perceived themselves at risk of AIDS (57 per cent) were more likely to report changing behaviour; they were also more likely to be infected with HIV. Other factors associated with behaviour change included having known someone with AIDS, having discussed AIDS with a male partner, and believing condoms are not dangerous.

Much evidence suggests that the feeling of being 'at risk' is actually associated with the level of medically accurate knowledge of the disease (Caprara *et al.*, 1993) and education status (Kronenfeld *et al.*, 1993). Feelings of vulnerability, therefore, are not reliable, objective indicators of either levels of high risk behaviour or contextual determinants of risk. In addition, behavioural change does not necessarily come about due to feelings of vulnerability. For example, Kigaru *et al.* (1993) questioned almost 4,000 adults in Nigeria and reported that 63 per cent had 'changed their lifestyle' due to AIDS, whereas only 11 per cent considered themselves to be at risk of infection. This apparent contradiction could be explained by the fact that feelings of vulnerability are

DO YOU THINK THERE IS ANY THREAT OF YOU GETTING AIDS?

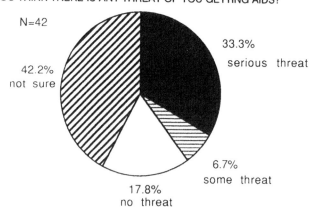

Figure 6.2. Perceived vulnerability to AIDS amongst secondary school students at Mpolweni Mission, Natal

reduced *as a consequence* of behavioural change, but this was not specified in the survey. In any case, there is no guarantee that the behavioural changes adopted by individuals, so inducing feelings of invulnerability, actually reduce their objective risk of infection. In Kwazulu/Natal, results of the KAPB survey of secondary school students at Mpolweni Mission conducted by the author reveal mixed levels of anxiety regarding HIV/AIDS (Figures 6.2 and 6.3), with one third of the students considering AIDS a 'serious threat' and almost a half consistently worrying about personal infection.

In the KAPB survey amongst students in the Oshakati area of Namibia, levels of concern are slightly higher. To the question 'Are you concerned about AIDS?', 61 (59.8 per cent) of respondents said yes, 24 (23.5 per cent) said no, and 17 (16.7 per cent) did not know or failed to answer the question. Seventy-two (70.6 per cent) claimed to have changed their behaviour with regard to AIDS. Of those, 27 (37.5 per cent) claimed to be using condoms, 40 (55.6 per cent) claimed to have reduced their number of partners, 1 (1 per cent) now abstains, and 4 (5.6 per cent) failed to answer. In relation to behavioural change, one respondent commented 'I had more than one girlfriend but now have completely changed my attitude about sex because of AIDS world-wide today; I do not sleep around any more' (male, 28). Conversely, comments such as the following are not atypical, 'no [I have not changed], because it did not attack me yet' (female,

DO YOU EVER WORRY THAT YOU COULD HAVE AIDS?

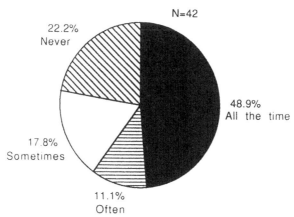

Figure 6.3. Anxiety regarding HIV infection

21). The subjective nature of the vulnerability is indicated further by the fact that infection levels amongst adolescents are probably slightly higher in the Natal sample compared to that in the Oshakati area. Exact figures do not exist, but HIV prevalence amongst Natal adolescents was estimated to be in the region of 5–10 per cent, whereas the figure for the Oshakati area was less than 5 per cent at the time of the fieldwork (Chapter 1).

Gaps in education are still evident and some misconceptions still persist, but overall the students are aware of the risks of infection. Levels of perceived vulnerability, however, are still not high enough to motivate behavioural change on a scale which is consistent enough to stop the spread of the virus. The reduction in the number of partners as a behavioural response, cited by 55.6 per cent of the Namibian students, for example, still indicates that there is only a limited reduction in high risk behaviour. Condom use is likely to be irregular and may depend on the particular choice of partner.

The health context of HIV/AIDS prevention

Explanation of the low level of priority accorded to AIDS through indicators of vulnerability is to be found in the context of people's lives. The male homosexual community in the United States responded extremely quickly to the AIDS epidemic once the infectious agent was recognised in the early 1980s. This was due primarily to the immediate prioritisation of AIDS in the lives of this community – it became the overriding health concern. Information was rapidly disseminated and the strength of the community networks was such that behavioural change was rapid and widespread (Panos, 1990). In sub-Saharan Africa, the prioritisation of the risk of HIV infection is often inhibited by feelings of fatalism due to other life-threatening conditions. An extreme, but pertinent example of this, is the case of truck and taxi drivers. The high mortality rates on some of the main truck and long distance taxi routes instils a feeling of *short term* survival for those who spend their lives on the roads. The high levels of infection in truck drivers and the prostitutes who cater for them are testament to this feeling of fatalism. An account of one trucker in Kenya exemplifies this:

> His logic is simple, he reckons the road will kill him before AIDS will. The highway death toll – over 300 in the last two months – reinforces this belief. The overturned lorries, the temporary liaisons, the transient lifestyle, the mirage of the truck city itself, all engender

a false sense of security and promote a short term, fatalistic view of life. (Cohen, 1993, p. 31)

In southern Africa, as discussed in Chapter 3, the disease has not been given the level of priority it has warranted, either at an institutional or individual level, partly due to prevailing structural conditions such as drought, economic restructuring and political instability. Non-prioritisation is also apparent with specific reference to health concerns. A national 1992 study by the Human Science Research Council (Conradie and Rabie, 1993) found through focus groups that tuberculosis, cancer, venereal disease, alcohol and drug abuse, unhygienic living conditions and measles were all given a higher priority than HIV/AIDS. In the research done by the author, conditions other than HIV/AIDS are accorded more attention by respondents in all but one of the field sites (Figure 6.4).

In the Bushbuckridge area of the former eastern Transvaal, for instance, the major health issue was water and sanitation, while focus group discussions also identified nutrition, kwashiorkor (a disease in children related to malnutrition), typhoid, diarrhoea, bilharzia (a water-borne infection of parasitic worms), measles, hypertension, tuberculosis, alcoholism, sexually transmitted disease and the lack of child care as prevalent health priorities.[1] Across the field sites, the major health concerns were perceived to be respiratory disease such as tubercu-

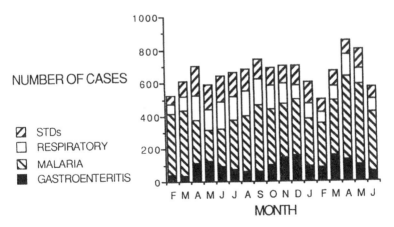

Figure 6.4. Primary health problems, Okatana Roman Catholic Hospital OPD, February 1992 – June 1993
N.B. Figures relate to OPD patients aged 5 years and over.

Table 6.1. Major perceived health concerns in the field sites

Condition	Respondents mentioning condition (%)					
	Field Site*					
	1	2	3	4	5	Average
Tuberculosis	24.0	24.3	15.8	34.0	6.0	20.8
Gastro-enteritis	1.0	4.0	19.8	21.0	37.0	16.6
Hypertension	5.0	7.5	16.5	36.0	9.0	14.8
Headaches	12.0	6.0	12.4	27.0	9.0	13.3
Influenza	1.0	21.5	19.8	14.0	2.0	11.7
Malaria	2.0	–	–	–	55.0	11.1
Foot/leg problems	6.0	6.0	–	35.0	3.0	10.0
Asthma	–	5.0	7.4	1.0	35.0	9.7
AIDS	**4.0**	**25.2**	**4.1**	**1.0**	**4.0**	**7.7**
Eye problems	7.0	–	8.3	7.0	6.0	5.7
STDs	**12.0**	**1.9**	**3.3**	–	**6.0**	**4.6**
Colds	–	–	–	–	12.0	2.4
Water/sanitation	6.0	–	–	5.0	–	2.2
Epilepsy	–	–	–	4.0	5.0	1.8
Malnutrition	–	0.9	2.5	–	5.0	1.7
Alcoholism	–	7.5	–	–	–	1.5
Skin problems	–	5.6	0.8	–	1.0	1.5
Pollution	–	5.6	–	–	–	1.1
Measles	–	–	–	–	5.0	1.0

* Field sites: 1. Lebowa; 2. Soweto; 3. Mpolweni, Natal; 4. Efaye, Natal;
5. Okatana, Namibia

losis, asthma, and possibly also influenza, as well as gastro-enteritis (linked to poor water supply and sanitation conditions) and hypertension (*hi-hi*) of which headaches are a symptom. Malaria was of considerable concern only in the Namibian field site. What must be noted is the low position which both AIDS and STDs hold when the conditions are ranked according to their number of mentions (Table 6.1). The responses are to the question 'what is the biggest health problem in the community?'. Multi-answering was accepted.

The reliability of the responses as objective indicators of the health status of the communities, must, of course, be questioned,[2] but what is under review is the subjective health environment rather than its objective counterpart. For comparison, the official health status of the Okatana community can be reviewed using records from the Roman Catholic Mission Hospital at the site (Figure 6.4). The figures from the respondents relate closely to the numbers of medical conditions diagnosed at the out-patients department (OPD) at the hospital, where malaria, gastro-enteritis, respiratory disorders and STDs are identified as the primary health problems in the community.

Comparing perceptions against the number of diagnoses would suggest that the severity of STD infections was understated by the community (mentioned by 6 per cent of respondents), either due to the difficulties associated with self diagnosis of STD infection (especially amongst women) or because of the stigma which surrounds such infections.

As discussed in Chapter 5, AIDS is perceived to be a considerable health concern only in the Soweto field site, which is possibly due to increased information and awareness of the disease, rather than a considerably higher HIV prevalence or AIDS case rate. A major obstacle inhibiting the success of AIDS prevention programmes in rural areas especially, is the existing myriad of health concerns with which the communities are familiar. They are the conditions which are *visible* and *immediate* to most people. The latency period of HIV dictates that most infections remain unnoticed, and that the virus continues to spread silently. At the time of the above surveys (October 1992–July 1993), HIV prevalence in the field sites stood at approximately 3–6 per cent of the adult population (Chapter 1), and with the doubling time of the virus around 12 months,[3] HIV/AIDS has to be considered, in objective terms, as one of the major health threats in all the communities. Its low prioritisation is due to the nature of the threat, seemingly *distant*, in both space and time.

Is the expectation of widespread, sustained behavioural change in this health environment realistic? Even with knowledge of the disease, concerns remain focused on the short term and related to prevailing health conditions. It is likely that HIV/ AIDS will remain a low priority until either local medical, water and sanitation conditions are dramatically improved, so improving the health status in relation to preventable diseases, or until the AIDS death rate increases markedly, by which point HIV would be endemic within the community. The theme which is emerging is that appropriate responses to the epidemic must have a large component which targets the context of infection, that is they are *development* processes. These are exclusively medium or long term processes, but the virus is spreading rapidly over a shorter time scale. The short term problem of HIV infection is negated by the possibly long term solution which incorporates development initiatives. This dilemma is further illustrated by examining the economic context of HIV epidemiology, and the implications for AIDS prevention.

The economic context of AIDS prevention

It is arguable that economic conditions in southern Africa comprise the most severe constraint on behavioural change in relation to HIV infection and influences the degree of behavioural skills conceptualised in the Information, Motivation and Behavioural Skills Model. The short term nature of prioritisation is exemplified through economic coping mechanisms. The context of poverty impacts on the epidemiology of HIV in a number of ways:

Women are forced into situations where sex is commoditised. This can take the form of overt prostitution or covert liaisons within the category of 'transactional sex' (Chapter 4). The question remains whether economic stress affects the actual amount of sexual activity, through more frequent partner changes within a community (leading to widespread infection) or whether increased stress determines the actual choice of partners (leading to the concentration of infection within core groups).

Psychological attention on immediate needs diminishes the importance of illness and even death in the long term. 'Safe sex' therefore is considered as less important than in the context of an economically stable environment, where longer term perspectives can be viewed with realism. This is not to say that the amount of behavioural change is directly correlated with the economic status of an individual or population group, rather that the constraints are more severe in groups with low socioeconomic status. The differentiation in levels of behavioural change in groups of prostitutes according to socioeconomic status illustrates this clearly. Levels of condom use are consistently lower among the poorest sex workers.

Poverty means that less disposable income is available for the treatment (and prevention) of other more immediate health concerns, most crucially STDs. The relatively recent introduction of user-charges in some countries, as part of government expenditure reduction programmes, for example ESAPs, has exacerbated this problem.

These processes operating in reality combine to produce high risk situations, and partly explain the vulnerable position of women. Evidence from interviews with 100 women in Uganda stresses this point, as '75 per cent of the women interviewed stated that AIDS and STD can be avoided if women have economic independence; only 25 per cent did not require economic independence as a means of preventing AIDS and STD' (Kato, 1993). Similarly in Zambia, where

> through focus group discussions with young men, we learned that AIDS was not one of their main concerns. They were curious (rather than concerned) about the effects of alcohol, tobacco and cannabis, but above all they were worried about their economic situation. (Mouli, 1992, p. 20)

The direct connection between economic stress and HIV infection was noted in South Africa by Strebel (1992), following interviews with seropositive women in the Western Cape, where 'a striking feature of these black women living with AIDS was their lack of economic independence and security' (p. 52). These women were all unemployed themselves, and all had partners who were unemployed. A 29 year old female respondent in Moloro (in the Lebowan field site) summed things up by saying that 'you can't have sex without money'.

The non-prioritisation of HIV/AIDS as a consequence of economic stress is self-evident, but how can this aspect of vulnerability be addressed in prevention schemes? The mitigation of structural processes at a local level is extremely difficult to operationalise with any level of sustainability, as the underlying

processes creating economic stress are not addressed. The programmatic focus on 'wealth' as a primary factor would be the
generation of services and employment opportunities, but the
mechanisms by which this can be achieved are yet to be teased
out from the considerable quantities of prevention rhetoric. The
improvement of economic conditions at a local level requires
medium and long term development initiatives, combined with
an immeasurable change in gender relations, which itself could
be either a cause or consequence of economic change. The crucial
point is that of the behavioural aspects of female economic dependence upon men, and this lies at the heart of so many sexual
contacts in African contexts. Even a small increase in the income
of a woman may have a dramatic effect on the nature of her
relationship with her partner(s). A small personal income could
do more than simply reduce dependency on the wages of the
partner, it could also boost self-esteem and create a feeling of
having some control over circumstance.

The current debates surrounding land inheritance rights and
property laws for women (especially those following divorce, or
death of the husband, and the legalities of the control of the
products from agriculture; Vaughan, 1994) are also crucial, as
they are addressing the concept of material resource control,
which could have far-reaching empowerment implications.[4] In
other words, the crucial ethos of *ambiocontrol* is addressed (Chapter 2). This developmental aspect of AIDS prevention, primarily
through income generation and income control, has received very
little attention and appears as no more than sprinkled anecdotes
in the reports of wider prevention programmes which focus on
education. Williams and Ray (1993, p. 28) mention initiatives in
Zimbabwe where women own and control small plots growing
vegetables on a commercial scale, providing over 100 women
with a regular source of income: 'As a result, fewer women are
now dependent on selling sex at the beerhall to make ends meet.'
At Chikankata in Zambia, income generation has been encouraged in seropositive women by supplying wool for knitting, so
allowing for the production and selling of sweaters (Williams,
1990, p. 28). Similar income generation schemes are also anticipated for seropositive women in Soweto, through the Society for
AIDS Families and Orphans (SAFO), but limited funds have
inhibited consolidation of the schemes. The generally scant attention paid to the very important aspect of income generation is
symptomatic of the misconceptualisation of AIDS prevention and
examples of successful applications are few and far between. An

holistic prevention project should have income generation as one of its core themes, and one can only speculate as to reasons for the failure of prevention programmers to recognise economic dependency in females as being fundamental to their vulnerability to HIV infection.

The development context of AIDS prevention

In terms of the interaction between development processes and the HIV/AIDS pandemic, the dominant conceptual model had been the adverse impact of AIDS related demographic disturbance on economic growth at all geographical scales. The reconceptualisation of AIDS prevention in recent years has transformed HIV/AIDS into a development issue as well as a health issue. The reasons for this transformation relate to the realisation that contextual factors are major determinants of high risk behaviour in relation to HIV infection, and that the partial resolution of these contextual inhibitors of behavioural change are fundamentally development issues. With HIV/AIDS recognised as a disease symptomatic of underdevelopment, there is still the need to specify which development processes should be prioritised in terms of HIV/AIDS prevention, other than the rebuilding of the health service infrastructure, and to what extent they should be seen as supplementary to, or congruent with, short term interventions.

The restructuring of the health service has been top priority for the new Government of National Unity (GNU) in South Africa, and the direction of change is firmly towards decentralisation and primary health care (PHC).[5] A hierarchical structure is envisaged of a single National Health Authority (NHA), with Provincial Health Authorities (PHAs) and finally District Health Authorities (DHAs), numbering about 100, each having a catchment of approximately 200,000–750,000 people. The main responsibility for health care delivery will be with the DHAs, who will have as much financial and administrative autonomy as possible. The restructuring of the health service must be linked in with other development processes, and government rhetoric to date has acknowledged the need for such horizontal programmes.

Viewing health as a development issue is an important conceptual development, and its translation into legislation and policies at a local level is crucial. Perceived development priorities at a localised scale were assessed in the field sites, in order to provide the exact development contexts of both health service restructuring and AIDS prevention. The non-prioritisation of

Table 6.2. Perceived development priorities in the sample communities

| Development need | Respondents mentioning need (%) | | | | | |
| | Field Site* | | | | | |
	1	2	3	4	5	Average
Water/sanitation	20.0	–	3.45	0.0	55.0	25.7
Schools/education	5.0	16.8	8.2	51.0	14.0	19.0
Clinic/health care	4.0	7.5	18.6	32.0	32.0	18.8
Crèche	3.0	17.8	6.2	22.0	15.0	12.8
Clothing/food for poor	8.0	–	3.4	12.0	37.0	12.1
Road/transport	4.0	–	25.6	3.0	5.0	7.5
Recreation facilities	10.0	14.0	5.2	4.0	–	6.6
Welfare for orphans	6.0	20.5	–	1.0	–	5.5
Business development	3.0	11.2	2.8	9.0	1.0	5.4
Electricity	–	–	11.0	13.0	2.0	5.2
New church	8.0	–	6.9	5.0	2.0	4.4
Shop	10.0	–	10.3	1.0	–	4.3
Old people's home	–	16.8	–	3.0	–	4.0
Housing	3.0	9.3	–	3.0	1.0	3.3
Community hall	4.0	–	6.9	–	–	2.2
Agriculture	3.0	–	–	–	6.0	1.8
AIDS organisations	–	7.5	–	–	–	1.5
Clean-up operations	–	3.7	–	–	2.0	1.1
Health education	1.0	3.7	–	–	–	0.9
Bar	3.0	–	–	–	–	0.6

* Field sites: 1. Lebowa; 2. Soweto; 3. Mpolweni, Natal; 4. Efaye, Natal; 5. Okatana, Namibia.

HIV/AIDS is partly a function of the perceived severity of the general conditions of under-development, and mental attention is distracted from the perceived vulnerability to HIV infection. The question was asked 'If you had R10,000 (about £2,000) to spend for the benefit of the whole community, how would you spend it?'. Multi-answering was accepted, and the question was open-ended. The responses are summarised in Table 6.2.

Each community has its own specific development needs profile, with some concerns, such as education, health care and crèches, being common to all the sites. The respondents in the Soweto community emphasise welfare provision above all else, while water is the dominant concern in the Namibian site. It is interesting to note that awareness of the needs of orphans is relatively high in the Soweto community, possibly indicating the severity of the impending orphan problem in the urban areas. Two important development priorities in relation to AIDS prevention are water provision and health care services. Both have a direct impact on the health environment, helping to prioritise the risk of HIV infection, and both are possible to address in the short term (Figure 6.5). In South Africa, it is estimated that more than 12 million people do not have access to clean drinking water and 21 million do not have adequate sanitation (ANC, 1994).

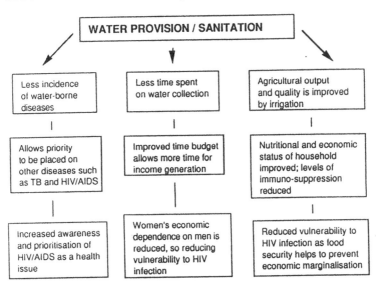

Figure 6.5. The linkages between water provision and HIV/AIDS prevention

Water and sanitation projects would contribute to HIV/AIDS prevention by prioritising AIDS as a health issue through the control of water related diseases such as gastro-enteritis, bilharzia and even malaria. The short term aims of the Reconstruction and Development Programme (RDP) were to 'provide all households with a clean, safe water supply of 20–30 litres per capita per day within 200 metres, an adequate/safe sanitation facility per site, and refuse removal system to all urban households'. The achievement of these goals in the short term would facilitate the prioritisation of HIV/AIDS at a household scale as other health and development issues are reduced in severity. Medium and long term goals are far more ambitious in relation to water provision, and no specific time references are given. In most rural communities, potable water is the central need and development efforts should be oriented around this. Improved time budgets resulting from water provision should improve income earning opportunities while improved agricultural output would have a number of economic and health benefits.

A separate development issue is that of recreation facilities. Several respondents made the direct link between the lack of facilities and the high teenage pregnancy rates (indicating that the adolescents are 'bored'), independent of other factors such as the different social and moral values found both within and between the sample communities (Chapter 4). Recreation facilities could be an important component of AIDS prevention strategies, especially in urban areas (Figure 6.6).

The issue of recreation facilities has already been identified by the Progressive Primary Health Care Network (PPHCN) and such facilities as table-tennis and volleyball equipment have been delivered and are being utilised in the Mapulaneng area of former Lebowa, for example.

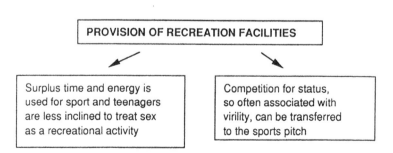

Figure 6.6. Recreation and HIV/AIDS prevention

The crucial point in relation to development priorities is that programmes which address issues of water, agriculture, income generation and transport improvement, to name a few, will have social effects which will reduce the vulnerability of people to HIV infection. Development programmes can supplement the short term technical interventions which focus on education, condom provision and STD treatment. The link has to be made between people's behaviour as a matter of individual volition, and people's behaviour as a necessary response to socio-environmental conditions. This leads us to the oft-mentioned buzz phrase 'empowerment'.

Prevention Through Empowerment

The link between context and the individual can be conceptualised as the process of empowerment, which is the provision of the ability to take control of a situation, to provide a sense of *ambiocontrol* and reduce vulnerability to HIV infection. With AIDS prevention, two themes emerge: that of behavioural empowerment, and structural empowerment. The term 'empowerment' is most often (but not exclusively) applied with specific reference to women:

- 'Behavioural empowerment' allows girls and women to have more control over their sexual activity, either through resisting sexual advances or through negotiating safe sex. It is the increase in the decision making ability of the women, so rendering them less vulnerable to infection, as the incidence of unsafe sex is reduced.

- 'Structural empowerment' is the reduction of economic dependence on men, and the improvement of women's sociolegal status (see above).

The problem lies in how this empowerment can be effected, as it is essentially a development issue. Behavioural empowerment is extremely problematic in many contexts as giving women, and young girls in particular, the ability to negotiate sexual activity contradicts many cultural mores. A condom is only as useful as the man's (as well as the woman's) willingness to use it, and that use will be largely dependent on the effectiveness of the local short term interventions, while the position of the women may be dependent on the effectiveness of the longer term interventions. The incremental empowerment of women in the spheres of law and economic production, however, has faced resistance, and programmes must be wary of accusations of cultural arrogance. This debate is somewhat acute in Zimbabwe, where President Mugabe outraged progressives and women's groups by condemning empowerment initiatives:

> If these ideas are being brought by whites amongst you as they come from Europe, they are bringing you terrible ideas. If the woman wants property in her own right, why did she get married in the first place? Better not wed then, because marriage means you are together with the husband as the head of the family.[6]

Structural and cultural inertia of this type will make the implementation of empowerment processes extremely problematic, inhibiting any widespread changes in the position of women in the short term. Symptomatic of this inertia is the broadening of behavioural empowerment strategies, which are increasingly targeting younger children, and the 'girl-child' in particular. The 5–14 age group is now termed the 'window of hope' group, as sexual activity has not yet commenced, and intervention strategies are looking to reach this group in order to have (positive) influence over sexual behaviour in adolescence.

Education strategies are also important in older age cohorts. Mouli (1992) argues that high risk situations can be mitigated by creating a social environment where high risk sexual behaviour is made more difficult by it being viewed as unacceptable. Douglas Feldman has a similar concept of 'value utilisation and norm change' in effecting behaviour change through the understanding of what local and age specific cultural factors determine the values and norms associated with sexual behaviour in adolescents (Feldman et al., 1995).

The argument that the prioritisation of AIDS requires a combination of both short term and long term interventions is nothing new, but what needs developing are the practical implications of this merger of time frames. The gulf between development programmes and AIDS prevention initiatives is immense in terms of coordination and funding horizons, and as Lucas (1992) stresses, 'we still need to find ways of convincing those involved in other development programmes of the need to address HIV as part of their programmes before the impact of sickness and death create a crisis'.

The fact that development programmes and AIDS prevention programmes do, in effect, have the same goals, has had little impact in terms of policy. There is the need to strengthen those areas of development programmes and development thinking which the social epidemiology of HIV/AIDS has shown to be weak, and possibly define and reduce in size the programmes that are specific to HIV. The sense of urgency and need for close coordination, especially in reference to the monitoring and evaluation of programmes is still lacking:

> Development programmes should now as a matter of course be judged by whether they decrease vulnerability to HIV infection – does this programme change gender relationships? Does it increase choices for women? Will it increase migration? (Lucas, 1992)

The shift in health spending by large international organisations towards multi-sectoral programmes is encouraging in this respect. Agencies such as the World Bank, the United States Agency for International Development (USAID), the Swedish International Development Authority (SIDA), UNESCO, UNICEF and the UNDP to name a few, are increasing their funding for health and AIDS projects, but still the interaction between development projects *per se* and AIDS prevention programmes is lacking. The creation of a Joint UN Programme on HIV/AIDS – 'UNAIDS' – which in effect merges the programmes of the World Bank, WHO, UNDP, UNICEF, UNESCO and the United Nations Population Fund (UNFPA) under a single activity umbrella, hopefully heralds an era of closer interaction between agencies and better coordination in relation to development initiatives and AIDS prevention. The precise coordination roles and functions of UNAIDS at a national scale however are still to be clarified and there is still much scepticism and ambivalence towards the replacement for the Global Programme on AIDS.

The Scales of Intervention

The mitigation of structural constraints at a local level, through the empowerment of agents and the instilling of an ethos of *ambiocontrol*, lies at the heart of AIDS prevention. At what scale this mitigation should be attempted is a crucial question, and experience has led analysts to the conclusion that to construct an intervention at anything beyond the community scale is inviting failure. The realities of conditions in many parts of rural South Africa dictate that planning and coordination of programmes have to be at a localised scale, due to the lack of resources and communications infrastructure. Large scale national programmes are often ill devised, with little or no targeting within the education messages, and are hampered by a host of restrictions which are moral, logistical and financial (Chapter 3). The intensity of education and efforts at facilitating behavioural change is such that a small scale of intervention is almost essential. The logistics of prevention dictate this:

The monitoring and evaluation of prevention initiatives can be undertaken only in relatively closed conditions, where the operating variables can be identified as far as possible. A successful programme can be recognised as such, with the important components easily identifiable. Translation of the programme into a different context is therefore possible.

Budgetary restrictions on prevention programmes often limit their operational scale. Analysis of the cost-effectiveness of interventions concludes that small scale interventions are more expensive per contact than programmes with a wide scale audience, but that this has to be balanced against that increased intensity of the contact.

The high degree of variability in both the objective and subjective health contexts between communities dictates that programmes have to be community specific when formulated (Chapters 4 and 5). A blanket approach cannot overcome these contextual differences as what may work in one place may not work in another. The concept of target groups is still crucial in intervention initiatives.

The perceptions of communities regarding the causes of social malaise and sexual behaviour, STDs and HIV/AIDS are internalised. The community is the scale of reference for the identification of cause and effect, even if the objective nature of the determinants (for example poor health services and poverty) are wide scale (Chapter 4). They are interpreted and acted upon at a local scale, within the spatial references of single communities (Butchart and Seedat, 1990).

Success can breed distortion. Many NGOs are suited to one scale only, and a successful programme developed and implemented at a community scale can be brought into disrepute through increased funding and subsequent expansion, as the original brief and scale of reference is exceeded. This could be applied to the successful TASO (The AIDS Service Organisation) project in Uganda (Klouda, 1992).

Successes in prevention have been almost exclusively at small socio-geographic scales. The approaches now being adopted, such as peer education strategies and home based care programmes require the *localisation* of the epidemic, as they need local coordination and the use of locally recognised individuals and organisations. For example, home based care programmes in Tanzania are having the effect of reducing stigmatisation within the communities, as the condition of patients are being seen to improve by the community members themselves (Flint, 1994). Home based care programmes are now being instituted in Kwazulu/Natal and are proving, with modification, to be cost effective at the present time[7] (Stewart, 1993).

Community participation is essential in the programmes, although this has proved to be logistically difficult to effect in some cases (Seeley *et al.*, 1992). In South Africa, the PPHCN, in particular, has been very active in encouraging schoolchildren to participate in World AIDS Day celebrations, which occur annually on 1 December. In former Lebowa, children wrote and performed songs, drew pictures and acted out plays in front of each other and their parents as part of the celebrations. In Kwazulu/Natal, schoolchildren act out plays with AIDS prevention messages in a wide scale programme under the auspices of the Dramaide (Drama in AIDS Education) project, pioneered at the University of Natal. The drama groups focus on the schools as the centre-points of each community, from where parents are encouraged to participate in the 'project day' (usually a Saturday) which is open to the whole community. The community, as a scale of both reference and intervention, is a crucial concept in AIDS prevention, and must remain the unit of analysis for the evaluation of both short and long term initiatives.

As coping with the epidemic becomes an important institutional priority, more emphasis will be placed on the community as the scale of intervention and coordination, as funds at the regional and national levels prove to be insufficient to provide institutional welfare at a formal level. This is one of the *raisons d'être* of home based care initiatives, but it also reflects the crucial role to be played by informal community structures such as rotating credit schemes, burial societies, and the fundamental ethos of community reciprocity, which is only partly compromised by the stigma associated with HIV/AIDS (Chapter 5). Networks of coping which are much in evidence in central Africa must also be present in southern Africa, and will soon be utilised in South Africa. These networks must be formally identified, with ways of integrating them into formal coping and prevention programmes investigated. This is most urgent in the case of the provision of welfare for AIDS orphans (Chapter 5).

The Future of HIV/AIDS in South Africa

The construction and development of appropriate AIDS prevention programmes will take place in a context which increasingly feels the impact of the epidemic. Peter Doyle[8] has produced the most credible of many projections of the epidemic in South Africa. This is summarised in Table 6.3.

The epidemic is predicted to peak at HIV prevalence of 27 per cent of the sexually active population by the year 2010, in the absence of behavioural change (Scenario 60). The model has recently been revised using data from the national HIV surveys of antenatal clinic attenders conducted by the former Department of National Health and Population Development (Chapter 1), resulting in Scenario 80. This projects the number of HIV infected at around 2,600,000 with a total of around 416,000 deaths by the year 2000. The demographic and socioeconomic implications of these figures are very serious, and it is still not fully understood how implementation of the post-apartheid Reconstruction and Development Programme will be affected by the epidemic. The literature on the impact of AIDS in South Africa is considerable and only a summary of projections is possible here:

• By the fiftieth year of the epidemic, the proportion of 15–25 year olds within the population structure will have doubled to around 33 per cent, with only 15 per cent of the population aged over 25, compared to 30 per cent at present (Rowley et al., 1990). This has adverse implications for the dependency ratio and the amount of available skilled labour. The socio-cultural consequences of such a demographic restructuring can only be guessed at.

Table 6.3. The Doyle Model of the AIDS epidemic in South Africa

	1991	1995	2000	2005
HIV infected				
Scenario 60[a]	97,000	970,000	4,112,000	6,410,000
Scenario 61[b]	97,000	970,000	3,700,000	4,762,000
Scenario 80[c]	80,816	756,237	2,606,517	4,509,870
AIDS sick				
Scenario 60	1,190	25,000	259,000	743,000
Scenario 61	1,190	25,000	255,000	618,000
Scenario 80	834	19,820	172,835	468,788
AIDS deaths				
Scenario 60	1,350	23,000	203,000	525,000
Scenario 61	1,350	23,000	197,000	429,000
Scenario 80	950	17,987	131,546	331,966
Cumulative deaths				
Scenario 60	2,200	47,000	602,000	2,588,000
Scenario 61	2,200	47,000	594,000	2,321,000
Scenario 80	950	36,000	416,000	1,660,000

a Scenario 60: HIV infection calibrated to data from other African countries.
b Scenario 61: HIV infection with the assumption of significant changes in sexual behaviour occurring 12 years into the epidemic.
c Scenario 80; Revised version of the Scenario 60 model using more recent data.
Sources: Doyle, 1993 and *Epidemiological Comments*, Vol. 20, No. 11, 1993.

• There is likely to be a reduction in the total fertility rate (TFR) as the increased maternal mortality rate means that fewer children are being born per woman. The overall dependency ratio will probably rise but not significantly, due to a rising infant mortality rate through paediatric AIDS. In Zambia the TFR is estimated to drop by about 5–10 per cent while the under five mortality rate will *increase* by around 10 per cent.

• Due to its efficient transport system and high mobility of labour, South Africa may see the lowest rural–urban differential in infection rates in sub-Saharan Africa.

• There is likely to be a shortage of skilled personnel, but unlikely to be any shortage of unskilled labour power. The economic implications for vocational training and medical costs for companies are ominous, and AIDS is now being considered as a cost factor of production.

• The cumulative number of AIDS orphans in South Africa was 20,000 in 1994 and will be approximately 531,000 by 2000 (Doyle, 1993; Fleming, 1994a).

• The direct medical costs of the epidemic will be beyond the scope of current health services. Estimates of costs vary from R6bn to R90bn in 2000. The range of estimates indicates the difficulties involved in planning the future of health service provision and allocation. Broomberg *et al.* (1993) estimate that cumulative direct costs of the epidemic will be between R15–30bn by 2000.

These implications of the epidemic are extremely severe, and the impact of AIDS is already being felt in countries immediately to the north. In Zambia, where antenatal HIV prevalence in Lusaka is in the region of 28 per cent (Chapter 1), AIDS is having an adverse effect on labour levels. In 1992, there was a crude death rate of 1.6 per cent in a sample of industries in Lusaka, with the figure projected to be 2.1 per cent for 1993 (Baggaley *et al.*, 1993). While AIDS is starting to have an impact in the former Frontline States, the question must be asked whether AIDS prevention policies in South Africa in the short term are responding to the projections. A National AIDS Plan for South Africa has been drawn up by the GPA, the

Centre for Disease Control and USAID, under the chairman-
ship of Dr Malcolm Steinberg (Fleming, 1994b; NACOSA,
1994). Three broad objectives are outlined:

• to prevent HIV transmission

• to reduce the personal and social impact of HIV infection

• to mobilise and unify national, provincial, international and
  local resources

These objectives are commendable, and the annual budget of
such a programme has been put at R256.77m, over ten times
that of the former Department of National Health and Population Development (Chapter 3). International support is now
readily available as South Africa has rejoined the World Health
Organization, and therefore can receive the full support of
UNAIDS, instituted in South Africa in January 1996. The
GPA had expressed confidence in the new administration and
'believes firmly that the epidemic can be curbed ... if South
Africa can implement the full range of interventions aimed at
reducing the sexual transmission of HIV'.[9] The commitment of
the political parties in addressing the epidemic has been questioned, but Dr Nkosazana Zuma, the Minister of Health, has to
date received the full support of most key actors in the epidemic, although her purported role in the Sarafina II scandal
in early 1996 has no doubt damaged her credibility.

The crucial issue in the future of the epidemic in South
Africa is the degree to which the disease is prioritised, not
only by the new government, but also by local and international NGOs and the private sector within South Africa. The
epidemic is at the stage where only immediate, comprehensive
action, involving education, extensive condom marketing (both
social and private), social development programmes and a massive restructuring of the health services will have any significant impact on the spread of HIV. Already, the priorities of
the new administration are fairly clear. Within the National
Health Authority, the priority programme is the restructuring
of the health service, and there is no guarantee that user
charges will not be implemented for medical care, which could
adversely impact on health seeking behaviour. Will enough
funds be made available for an intensive education campaign
and a STD control programme?[10] Zuma seemed confident that

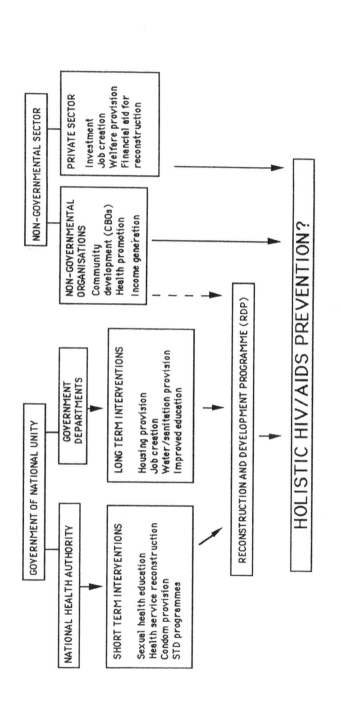

GOVERNMENT OF NATIONAL UNITY

NATIONAL HEALTH AUTHORITY

GOVERNMENT DEPARTMENTS

SHORT TERM INTERVENTIONS

Sexual health education
Health service reconstruction
Condom provision
STD programmes

LONG TERM INTERVENTIONS

Housing provision
Job creation
Water/sanitation provision
Improved education

NON-GOVERNMENTAL SECTOR

NON-GOVERNMENTAL ORGANISATIONS

Community development (CBOs)
Health promotion
Income generation

PRIVATE SECTOR

Investment
Job creation
Welfare provision
Financial aid for reconstruction

RECONSTRUCTION AND DEVELOPMENT PROGRAMME (RDP)

HOLISTIC HIV/AIDS PREVENTION?

Figure 6.7 *opposite* Conceptual model of the future of AIDS prevention in South Africa

---

at least R100m could be spent on AIDS prevention in 1994–95, with over half of this coming from foreign donors.[11] An encouraging sign is that the National AIDS Plan (NAP) is to be managed as part of the RDP, so facilitating inter-departmental coordination, as the AIDS epidemic must be treated as more than a medical/health issue if prevention measures are to have any chance of success. The priorities of the government as a whole may themselves prove to be essential components of a complete AIDS prevention programme. The ANC manifesto documented the social development programme:[12]

- to provide jobs and training for 2.5 million unemployed over ten years

- build 1 million homes within the next five years

- provide running water and toilets for 1 million families in five years

- supply electricity to 2.5 million homes in five years

- double the number of free school text books within a year

These programmes would complement an AIDS prevention programme to provide a context allowing for the prioritisation of AIDS (Figure 6.7). The participation of NGOs and the private sector is crucial in the prevention effort, and the government is still trying to incorporate NGOs into the RDP without being seen to usurp both their influence at a local level and, more importantly, their funding base from abroad. The government is now in competition with the estimated 50,000 NGOs in South Africa for external funding, and there are some indications that the government, while recognising the importance of NGO activities, is attempting to regulate and determine NGO activity as a precondition for their participation in the RDP.[13]

The action of the government and NGOs must be complemented by the private sector, which will be badly affected by the epidemic in a number of ways:

- The workforce will not decline but it will change in structure, being more youthful, inexperienced and less well trained. Labour and retraining costs will rise and medical costs will spiral.

- There could be a disproportionately high number of losses amongst the skilled workforce. Experience from the rest of Africa has shown that this segment of the workforce is often the first to be affected (Ainsworth and Over, 1992).

- Absenteeism caused by AIDS related illnesses will be more financially damaging in the long term than the loss of the workers through death. Employees will require more time off to attend funerals and absenteeism will increase when workers, or even the relatives of the workers, are sick.

- Lowered productivity will result, as the syndrome is characterised by recurrent bouts of ill-health.

- Ostracisation at the workplace of people who are HIV-positive will affect morale and performance.

- As well as the direct impacts there will also be indirect effects, such as the drop in consumer spending as the economic effects of AIDS spreads throughout society.

The private sector can respond to the epidemic and supplement wider scale prevention programmes, through its own, possibly company-specific, workplace AIDS policies. Policies include the provision of free or low cost condoms, and there are NGOs already active in this respect, such as the Population Services International organisation. The social marketing of condoms in *shebeens* or *spaza* shops can be undertaken by encouraging existing entrepreneurial networks, while indirect intervention can take the form of extending networks with smaller businesses and encouraging economic development at a grass roots level.

Priorities and Prevention

The realistic prospects of curbing the HIV/AIDS epidemic in South Africa are, however, minimal. The virus is spreading at such a pace, with an estimated 500 new infections every day, that an holistic programme will be in place far too late to have any impact on the epidemic. Despite governmental rhetoric, the non-prioritisation of AIDS will remain for years to come, as the concerns of welfare, housing, employment and social problems such as crime, in particular, dominate both politics and community life. The situation is strikingly similar in Namibia, where post-independence reconstruction has failed to have a major impact on development indicators. Recent reports from Soweto emphasise these concerns, with community mobilisation around the improvement of relations with the police. The president of the Soweto Civic Association, Isaac Mogase, was reported as saying at a rally,

> We used to say 'police out of the townships', but now it's criminals we want out. It is the most important thing for the people, ending crime, and we are going to hold events like this all over Soweto.[14]

Similar sentiments were expressed by a civic worker at the rally:

> Fighting crime is the most important thing for us. I will tell you why. Even if you have a perfect education system, the hooligan and criminal element will continue to disrupt classes. If you try and build houses, the criminals will steal the materials. When the electricity workers come, we have to give them protection otherwise the criminals steal their vehicles. Last week two Telkom workers were shot dead with AK-47s.

The political struggle has been replaced with the anticipation of change at ground level. It will take a long time before these hopes are realised, and the series of strikes in July and August 1994 (most notably that of 25,000 car workers) indicates that patience will not be maintained indefinitely. Given the rapid political change in South Africa, the illusion must not be given that there has been, or will be rapid contextual change. The conditions and macro-processes which operated to deprioritise the epidemic at the institutional level are still in existence – migrant labour flows, poor health conditions, social instability (though slightly depoliticised in character), high levels of unemployment and social mores are still in existence. The RDP, if it survives as a programme, is a long term strategy, which may not have any actual effect on the course of the epidemic for another five years. In the short term, interventions can be put in place and those already in existence stepped up and consolidated, in order to save as many lives as possible. The increased support of the private sector is vital in this regard. Positive moves now, however, will be instituted many years too late to have any significant impact, and expectations that the epidemic will be curbed will prove to be unfounded. Nowhere in sub-Saharan Africa has a NACP significantly changed the course of the epidemic, and this, unfortunately, will also be the case in South Africa. The hope remains that the impacts of AIDS are foreseen and prepared for. The success of post-apartheid reconstruction depends on this response to the epidemic, the full implications of which will soon affect individuals, communities, and the state alike.

Notes and References

1. The HIV/AIDS Epidemic in Southern Africa

1. UNAIDS Fact sheet, July 1996, Geneva.
2. Reported by the Panos Foundation in *AIDS Analysis Africa* (Southern African Edition) vol. 6, no. 6, April/May 1996.
3. UNAIDS, Fact sheet, July 1996.
4. The bibliography of the Network of AIDS Researchers in Eastern and Southern Africa (NARESA) in April 1993 lists just seven articles, two of which are news items.
5. The literature on this aspect of AIDS is vast. References cited in the following sections are the most accessible in academic terms and tend to be review articles. The work by Mann, Tarantola and Netter (1992) is the main reference for much of the information.
6. Dr Anthony Fauci, reported from the International AIDS Conference in Amsterdam, 1992, Reuters, 23 July 1992.
7. See 'How HIV-related opportunistic infections vary around the world', in *The AIDS Report* (editorial), 1994, Fall, pp. 3–7.
8. This may not be necessarily true if HIV crosses the placenta independently of a fluid medium.
9. Reported in *Epidemiological Comments*, vol. 20, no. 11, 1993, p. 198.
10. For a review of recent research in this area see Webb, D. and Fleming, A. (1996) The essential role of antenatal clinics in AIDS control, *Current AIDS Literature*, May 1996.
11. Reported in *Nature*, Vol. 369, 1994, p. 429.
12. Professor Alan Fleming, personal communication.
13. *WorldAIDS*, March 1992, p. 11.
14. Reuters, 2 October 1991.
15. The use of the oral contraceptive pill may be misinterpreted as a risk factor *per se* as it may indicate a non-defined behavioural factor, i.e. a high number of partners.

16. The exact reasons for this are not quite clear, but could relate to the low amount of sexual interaction between the core groups and the general population, the low presence of STDs which facilitate transmission, or the increased amount of 'safer' sexual behaviour.

17. See *AIDS Captions*, Vol. 1, No. 3, 1994, which concentrates on AIDS in Asia.

18. Reported in the *Natal Witness*, 13 May 1993.

19. See 'Returnees aggravate Mozambican HIV situation', in *AIDSLINK*, No. 20, September 1995, p. 1.

20. *WorldAIDS*, July 1994, p. 9.

21. Figures from the Ministry of Health, Gaborone, reported in *AIDS Analysis Africa*, Vol. 6, No. 3, June 1996.

22. 'Sex-for-release at border post', *The Namibian*, 4 February 1994.

23. *Frontlines*, No. 3, 1995.

24. Figures from the NACP, presented to the SANASO Conference in Maputo in July 1994.

25. Figure reported to the World Health Organization, from the NACP.

26. Reported in *The Namibian*, 17 June 1994.

27. *The Namibian*, 2 April 1993.

2. Conceptualising HIV Epidemiology

1. Jonathan Mann, reported in the *Guardian*, 24 April 1992.

2. Reprinted in *AIDS Analysis Africa (Southern African Edition)* Vol. 3, No. 1, p. 6.

3. 'High risk behaviour' can be defined as anything which can possibly cause the transmission of HIV, but usually relates to sexual promiscuity, or sexual contact with assumed 'high risk' persons, such as prostitutes, and is most often characterised by the lack of condom use.

4. David Hume, essentially an empiricist philosopher, in that he claimed that all reason is dependent on experience, posited that the implication of causation between two events is not justified by observation alone, and that there are no rational grounds for assuming repetition of future events on simple observation of a single, discrete event (such as a billiard ball moving when struck by another) or repeated events in the present.

5. Some scientists in Nairobi were reported to have discovered

possible 'immunity' to HIV amongst some prostitutes in the city. *The Guardian*, 19 October 1993.

6. Health Services Development Unit, Acornhoek, 1992, unpublished data.

7. Much of the information that follows is derived from unpublished surveys conducted by the Health Services Development Unit, Acornhoek.

8. Sylvia Mafu, Noodberg Clinic, personal communication.

9. The principal of the village school, who assisted in the formulation of the fieldwork, is the nephew of Harry Gwala, a prominent ANC leader in Natal.

10. *The Sunday Times Magazine*, 27 March 1994, p. 5.

3. The Political Economy of AIDS in Southern Africa

1. *Southern African Economist*, Vol. 5, No. 2, p. 7, April 1992.

2. *AIDS Analysis Africa*, May/June 1991, p. 6.

3. Katele Kalumba, personal communication.

4. *Critical Health*, 22, April 1988, p. 20.

5. 'Apathy affects condom sales', *Weekly Mail and Guardian*, 31 March 1995.

6. *Mail and Guardian*, 9–14 March 1996.

7. 'Lack of funds leads to AIDS test cut', *The Star* (Johannesburg), 30 August 1994.

8. See 'Southern African NGOs seize the initiative', *WorldAIDS*, November 1990, pp. 5–7.

9. Dr Marian Seabrook, Campus Health, University of the Witwatersrand, personal communication.

10. Claire Fleming, Coordinator of SAFO, personal communication.

11. AIDSCOM (US$24m, 1987–92) is a large project within US-AID's AIDS Technical Support Project, which 'has helped organisations apply communication and behavioural sciences to AIDS and has assisted in developing institutional capacities for health communication efforts' (Mann, Tarantola and Netter, 1992, p. 803).

12. Interview with Dr Izak Fourie, Medical Advisor to the Chamber of Mines, August 1992.

13. *The Economist*, 23 April 1994.

14. 'Freedom in SA fails to bring relief from crime', *The Independent*, 4 August 1994.

15. 'Township blanks out its horror', *The Independent*, 16 February 1994.

16. 'Township shooting leaves 11 dead', *The Times*, 7 July 1994.
17. *Weekly Mail and Guardian*, 5–11 May 1995.
18. *The Money Programme*, BBC 2, 31 May 1992.
19. This point was emphasised many times by respondents during discussions, but blatantly portrayed in an AIDS education play written and staged by school students in Natal, in which 'Freddy Mercury enters with music playing in the background. He is dancing with a girl who he propositions. He tells the audience that he has many girlfriends and boyfriends. The girl leaves and a boy enters, very camp, and tells Freddy how much he loves him and they leave the stage together' (from the Documentation of DRAMAIDE, University of Natal, Pietermaritzburg, unpublished).
20. *The Star* (Johannesburg), 26 November 1992.
21. *Natal Witness*, 13 May 1993.
22. *The Star* (Johannesburg), 30 November 1992.
23. Calculations made by the South African Reserve Bank, reported in the *Natal Witness*, 13 May 1993.
24. *The Star* (Johannesburg), 14 August 1992.
25. *The Sunday Times* (London), 14 June 1992.
26. *Business Day*, 19 January 1993.
27. *Daily Telegraph*, 6 March 1992.
28. *The Star* (Johannesburg), 14 August 1992.
29. Interview with Dr Malcolm Steinberg, Director of the MRC (Cape), January 1993.
30. Interview with Dr Izak Fourie, Medical Advisor to the Chamber of Mines, August 1992.
31. *Critical Health*, 22, April 1988, p. 14.
32. Interview with Dr Izak Fourie, Medical Advisor to the Chamber of Mines, August 1992.
33. Ron Ballard, South African Institute for Medical Research, personal communication.
34. Tintswalo Hospital report, March 1992.
35. Community Practice Project, Health Services Development Unit.
36. Reported in *The Namibian*, 17 March 1994.
37. Dr Maija Palander, a visiting Finnish STD specialist at Onandjokwe Hospital, personal communication.
38. The staff involved with blood collection believe that many donors give blood in order to discover their HIV status, so introducing a sample bias of 'higher risk' donors. If this were to be the case, a higher than expected percentage of HIV-positive donors would be donating for the first time. The

blood collection centres are visited relatively frequently by the mobile transfusion clinic, so most of the donors could have donated previously if they had so desired. However, out of a sample of 50 donors who tested HIV-positive, 23 (46 per cent) were first time donors, whereas of a sample of 117 donors who tested HIV-negative, 61 (52.1 per cent) were first time donors. Also the impression was given to the staff that many students wanted to give blood as they would be seen to be doing something positive for the community.

39. The correlation coefficient of determination is a figure between 0–1, 0 being a perfect non correlation (totally random), 1 being a perfect correlation.

40. Sister Salmi Imbondi, Oshakati State Hospital, Blood Transfusion Service, personal communication.

41. *AIDS Analysis Africa* (Southern Africa edition) October–November 1991.

42. HSDU (1992) Health situation analysis, unpublished, Acornhoek.

43. This mixture is also believed to be an aphrodisiac, and forms the basic ingredients of 'Spanish Fly' ointments. It is in fact highly toxic, possibly causing severe haemorrhaging and damage to the mucosal lining of the gut and urinary tract.

44. *Mozambiquefile*, No. 207, October 1993, p. 19.

45. Government of the Republic of Zambia/UN (1996) *Prospects for Sustainable Human Development in Zambia: More Choices for our People*, (self published).

4. The Behavioural Context of the HIV/AIDS Epidemic

1. Life worlds are the perceived environments of individuals which are unique to each individual. The perception of the life world is dependent on the daily activities and the way the individual interacts with other people and social phenomena.

2. Significance values, represented by p, indicate the likelihood of the observed association occurring by chance. The smaller the value of p, therefore, the stronger the degree of significance of the relationship, and the smaller the chance of the null hypothesis (H_0) being correct. I have generally used the 95 per cent significance level as a cut-off threshold.

3. This information was derived from a 28 year old respondent in Okatana who claimed that 'some girls try to get pregnant to get the fine of R800', which is payable to the girl's parents.

4. The amount of payment liable is decided by the *induna* and is applied if the *lobola* is not forthcoming from the male.
5. Deborah Tromp, Pietermaritzburg based 'Drama in AIDS Education' group, personal communication.
6. The main criterion for calculating the *lobola* is the woman's standard of education and therefore her earning power. My interpreter, at the time of the work, was seriously considering divorcing his wife because she was likely to fail her matric examinations. He is otherwise unemployed and says that he needs a wife with 'earning potential'.
7. Health Services Development Unit, Tintswalo Hospital, Acornhoek, unpublished data, 1991. N.B. standard 10 students can be in their late twenties, and this data would not preclude those over 20.
8. Shirley Ngwenya, Health Services Development Unit, Tintswalo Hospital, Acornhoek, personal communication.
9. Jonathan Stadler, Department of Social Anthropology, University of the Witwatersrand, personal communication.
10. The rates of adolescent and illegitimate pregnancy are arguably no higher in southern Africa than in the Western world, depending on the actual definition being used. Data from the 1991 census in the United Kingdom put rates of births 'out of wedlock' as high as 40 per cent of the total in some areas (*The Sunday Times*, 22 May 1994, p. 2); the figure is nearer 50 per cent in France. In Western societies such as Britain, the proportion of technically illegitimate children born to couples in permanent or semi-permanent relationships is relatively high: over 50 per cent according to the American sociologist Charles Murray (*Guardian*, 25 May 1994, p. 7). This is probably higher than in the southern African context, where pregnancies resulting from casual liaisons are far more numerous. Evidence for this, however, is anecdotal and there remains a dearth of reliable information on this issue.
11. HSDU, Health situation analysis, Acornhoek, 1992, unpublished.
12. The PPHCN is employing two field workers to provide education regarding STDs and AIDS to rural areas in New Hanover.
13. On my walks around the village I noticed many boys as young as 9 or 10 years old selling sweets and frozen drinks. Girls were to be found helping their mothers prepare food – any food the girls sold was on their mothers' behalf.
14. The main clients of the more overt local prostitutes are

employed men – the going rate per 'round' is R20–50. Being a *lekgowa* (white), I would be asked to pay R400, according to one 19 year old prostitute.
15. Sylvia Mafu, senior nurse at Noodsberg clinic, Dalton, New Hanover, personal communication.
16. UNICEF have estimated this imbalance as an adult female to male ratio of 2:1 (cited in Botelle, 1992, p. 30).
17. Quoted in the *Natal Witness*, 15 April 1993.
18. Medical superintendent, Monze District Hospital, personal communication.
19. Again this situation is reminiscent of current debates in the United Kingdom.
20. *Sunday Tribune*, 14 October 1990.
21. The term 'peri-urban' is used as this is the accepted terminology to describe these settlements in the Oshakati/Ondangwa nexus area. The communal areas of the north officially have no urban areas, but these definitions are under legislative review. 'Town' status has been granted on to Oshakati, for example, but the resultant changes are administrative only.

5. *Community Responses to HIV/AIDS*

1. This terminology is borrowed from Barnett and Blaikie (1992) who used these distinctions in relation to households. *Affliction*, in this sense, relates to the direct infection and condition of someone who is seropositive, while *affected* relates to those not personally infected but whose life world is integrally connected to someone who is, such as relative or work colleague.
2. *Epidemiological Comments*, Vol. 20, No. 11, November 1993, p. 187.
3. AIDS surveillance in Kwazulu, 1992, Alan Jaffe, personal communication.
4. Dr Maija Palander, personal communication.
5. The categorisation of status was in the response to the question 'are you married?' A negative response I have categorised as single, despite the possibility of the respondent being in a permanent or semi-permanent relationship. The distinction surrounds actual *conjugality*. As the claim for marriage is derived from the respondent, no distinction is made between 'traditional' or 'official' marriage.
6. On the occasion where the question was misunderstood, the

answer 'they will die' was often given. At these times the
question was repeated, with the emphasis on the appropriate
community response to that person.

7. Reported in *WorldAIDS*, No. 33, 1994, p. 3, and *The Economist*, 19 March 1994, p. 69.
8. Health Services Development Unit, Acornhoek, 1991, unpublished data.
9. The radio station concerned is apparently Radio Zulu, based
   in Durban. Reporting such as this contradicts so much positive information heard on the radio, and has to be considered
   as very dangerous, and not simply because of the confusion it
   creates.
10. 'No school for kids with AIDS', *Cape Times*, 9 August 1994.
11. Reported in *Africa Health*, January 1990, p. 7.
12. The Cuban system of segregation involves communes of peo-
    ple infected with HIV who are cared for under closed (and
    reputably quite comfortable) conditions. This method of iso-
    lation is well analysed in *AIDS & Society*, January/February
    1992.
13. The paper cited is unpublished to date.
14. *Africa Health*, March 1990, p. 6.
15. *Sunday Tribune*, 14 March 1993.
16. In this case 'orphan' is defined as a child below the age of 18,
    or who is still in school, who has lost one or both parents.

6. The Development of HIV/AIDS Prevention Programmes

1. Health Services Development Unit, unpublished data, 1992.
2. Problems may have arisen during the translation of the respondents' replies. This was minimised by the translators all
   having a basic medical knowledge (two translators employed
   were health workers), but the respondents' subjective descrip-
   tions of the conditions may have been misinterpreted by the
   translator.
3. *Epidemiological Comments*, Vol. 21, No. 4, April 1994.
4. For example, see 'Property-grabbing: why Zambia needs
   stronger laws to protect widow's rights', *AIDS Analysis
   Africa*, Vol. 4, No. 4, 1992, pp. 1–7.
5. The new policies are outlined in the RDP policy framework
   (ANC, 1994).
6. 'Long-running "war of sexes" hots up in Zim', *The Namibian*,
   2 September 1994.
7. As the AIDS case rate is still relatively low in Natal/Kwa-

zulu, compared to southern Zambia where the projects were pioneered, interaction and coordination with TB programmes in rural areas has been posited as the best way of developing the programme in the short term.

8. Chief Actuary for Metropolitan Life Association, Cape Town.
9. 'The World Health Organization and the New South Africa', *AIDS Analysis Africa*, (Southern Africa Edition) Vol. 5, No. 2, August/September 1994, p. 2.
10. 'AIDS plan not enough', *Business Day*, 2 July 1994.
11. 'Finally, the state gets serious about AIDS', *The Weekly Mail*, 22 July 1994.
12. *The Sunday Times*, 30 January 1994.
13. 'Licence plan to control RDP billions' and 'No-go unless NGOs deliver the goods', *The Weekly Mail and Guardian*, 26 August 1994; 'Stricter controls for NGOs', *The Weekly Mail and Guardian*, 23 September 1994.
14. 'Old foes in Soweto unite to fight crime', *The Independent*, 15 August 1994.

Bibliography

Abdool Karim, Q., Abdool Karim, S.S. and Nkomokazi, J. (1991) Sexual behaviour and knowledge of AIDS among urban black mothers, *South African Medical Journal*, Vol. 80, pp. 340–3.

Abdool Karim, Q., Abdool Karim, S.S., Singh, B. *et al.* (1992) Seroprevalence of HIV infection in rural South Africa, *AIDS*, Vol. 6, pp. 1535–9.

Abramson, P.A. (1992) Sex, Lies, and Ethnography, in Herdt, G. and Lindenbaum, S. *The Time of Aids*, pp. 101–23.

Ahrenson-Pandikow, H. (1992) *Survey of attitudes towards the use of contraceptives in Namibia*, Namibian Institute for Social and Economic Research, Research Report No. 15, University of Namibia, Windhoek.

African National Congress (1994) *The Reconstruction and Development Programme; a policy framework*, ANC, Johannesburg.

Agadzi, V.K. (1990) *AIDS: the African perspective of the killer disease*, Ghana Universities Press, Accra.

AIDS Analysis Africa (1993), In the black townships of South Africa – and if you are black – this is the reality of fighting AIDS, Vol. 3, No. 5, p. 1.

Ainsworth, M. and Over, M. (1992) *The economic impact of AIDS: shocks, response and outcomes*, The World Bank, Africa Technical Department, Population, Health and Nutrition Division, Technical Working Paper No. 1.

Akeroyd, A.V. (1994) HIV/AIDS in Eastern and Southern Africa, *Review of African Political Economy*, No. 60, pp. 173–84.

Anderson, R.M. (1991) Mathematical models of the potential impact of AIDS in Africa, in Piot, P. *et al.*, *AIDS in Africa*, pp. 37–44.

Anderson, R.M. and May, R.M. (1992) Understanding the AIDS Pandemic, *Scientific American*, May 1992, pp. 20–6.

Anderson, R.M., May, R.M., Bailey, M.C., Garnett, G.P. and

Rowley, J.T. (1991) The spread of HIV-1 in Africa: sexual contact patterns and the predicted demographic impact of AIDS, *Nature*, Vol. 352, pp. 581–9.

Andima, J., Kahuika, S. and Melber, H. (1994) *Population issues in Namibia*, Namibian Economic Policy Research Unit Working Paper No. 32, Windhoek.

Ankrah, E.M. (1989) AIDS: Methodological problems in studying its prevention and spread, *Social Science and Medicine*, Vol. 29, No. 3, pp. 265–76.

Antwi, P., Tipping, S., Kumah, O.M. *et al.* (1993) *AIDS awareness and high risk behaviour in Ghana: results of a national survey*, VIIIth International Conference on AIDS in Africa, Marrakesh, 1993.

Armstrong, S. (1993) The last taboo, *WorldAIDS*, No. 29, pp. 6–9.

Bagarukayo, H., Shuey, D., Babishangire, B. and Johnson, K. (1993) *An operational study relating to sexuality and AIDS prevention among primary school students in Kabale District of Uganda*, Amref, Entebbe.

Baggaley, R., Chilanga, D., Godfrey-Faussett, P. and Porter, J. (1993) Impact of HIV on Zambian businesses, VIIIth International Conference on AIDS in Africa, Marrakesh, 1993.

Baldo, M. and Cabral, A.J. (1990) Low intensity wars and social determination of the HIV transmission: The search for a new paradigm to guide research and control of the HIV/AIDS pandemic, in Stein, Z. and Zwi, A. *Action on AIDS in Southern Africa*, pp. 36–42.

Barnett, T. and Blaikie, P. (1992) *AIDS in Africa; its present and future impact*, Belhaven Press, London.

Barongo, L.R. (1992) The epidemiology of HIV-1 infection in urban areas, roadside settlements and rural villages in Mwanza Region, Tanzania, *AIDS*, Vol. 6, pp. 1521–8.

Bassett, M. (1993) Social and economic determinants of vulnerability to HIV infection: the Zimbabwe experience, *AIDS Analysis Africa*, July/August, pp. 9–11.

Bassett, M., Mbizvo, M.T., Ray, S. *et al.* (1993) *Separation from wife, high risk behaviour and HIV among male, urban workers in Harare, Zimbabwe*, VIIIth International Conference on AIDS in Africa, Marrakesh, 1993.

Berkley, S., Naamara, W., Okware, S. *et al.* (1990) AIDS and HIV infection in Uganda – are more women infected than men?, *AIDS*, Vol. 4, pp. 1237–42.

Borgdorff, M., Barongo, L.R., Van Jaarsveld, E. *et al.* (1993)

Sentinel surveillance for HIV-1 infection: how representative are blood donors, outpatients with fever, anaemia, or sexually transmitted diseases, and antenatal clinic attenders in Mwanza region, Tanzania? *AIDS*, Vol. 7, pp. 567–72.

Botelle, A. (1992) *Onaanda community-based road construction project, western Owambo region; a base line socio-economic survey*, Namibian Institute for Social and Economic Research, University of Namibia, Windhoek.

Botha, J.F., Ritchie, M.J.J., Dusheiko, G.M., Mouton, H.W.K. and Kew, M.C. (1984) Hepatitis B virus carrier state in black children in Ovamboland: role of perinatal and horizontal infection, *The Lancet*, 1984 (i) pp. 1210–11.

Botha, J.L., Bradshaw, D., Gonin, R. and Yach, D. (1988) The distribution of health needs and services in South Africa, *Social Science and Medicine*, Vol. 26, No. 8, pp. 845–51.

Broomberg, J. (1993) Current research on the economic impact of HIV/AIDS: a review of the international and South African literature, in Cross, S. and Whiteside, A., *Facing up to AIDS*, pp. 34–57.

Broomberg, J., Steinberg, M., Masobe, P. and Behr, G. (1993) The economic impact of the AIDS epidemic in South Africa, in Cross, S. and Whiteside, A. *Facing up to AIDS*, pp. 158–90.

Butchart, A. and Seedat, M. (1990) Within and without: images of community and implications for South African psychology, *Social Science and Medicine*, Vol. 31, No. 10, pp. 1093–1102.

Cadman, V. (1987) Gazankulu; land of refuge and relocation, *Indicator SA*, Vol. 4, No. 3, pp. 101–3.

Caldwell, J.C. and Caldwell, P. (1993a) The nature and limits of the sub-Saharan African AIDS epidemic: evidence from geographic and other patterns, *Population and Development Review*, Vol. 19, No. 4, pp. 817–48.

——(1993b) The South African fertility decline, *Population and Development Review*, Vol. 19, No. 2, pp. 225–62.

——(1996) The African AIDS epidemic, *Scientific American*, March 1996, pp. 62–8.

Cambell, I. (1990) Caring for people with AIDS: it can be done! *Africa Health*, July 1990, pp. 46–7.

Caprara, A., Seri, D., De Gregorio, G.C. *et al.* (1993) The perception of AIDS in the Béte and Baoule of the Ivory Coast, *Social Science and Medicine*, Vol. 36, No. 9, pp. 1229–35.

Carael, M., Cleland, J., Adeokun, L. *et al.* (1991) Overview and selected findings of sexual behaviour surveys, in Piot, P. *et al., Aids in Africa,* pp. 65–74.

Carswell, W. (1993) HIV in South Africa, *The Lancet,* Vol. 342, p. 132.

Catholic Diocese of Ndola, AIDS Department, (1995) *Prevalence of orphans and their education status in Nkwazi Compound – Ndola,* paper presented at the Zambian National AIDS Network Conference, Lusaka, May 1995.

Children in Distress Project (1991) *Enumeration and needs assessment survey for orphans in Matero East, Lusaka, Zambia,* Unpublished Report.

Chin, J. and Mann, J.M. (1988) The global patterns and prevalence of AIDS and HIV infection, *AIDS 2* (suppl. 1), pp. 247–52.

Chipfakacha, V. (1993) Prevention of sexually transmitted diseases; the Shurugwi sex-workers project, *South African Medical Journal,* Vol. 53, pp. 40–1.

Chisango, B., Chihwai, D. and Machamire, C. (1993) *Why there are new cases of STD/HIV despite the campaigns,* VIIIth International Conference on AIDS in Africa, Marrakesh, 1993.

Christie, G. (1991) AIDS in South Africa, *South Africa International,* July, 1991, pp. 23–7.

Cloke, P., Philo, C. and Sadler, D. (1991) *Approaching Human Geography,* Paul Chapman Press, London.

Cohen, D. (1993) Road to ruin, The *Guardian Weekend,* 11 December 1993, pp. 28–35.

Collins, P. (1990) *AIDS: political and economic considerations,* Department of Political Studies, University of Cape Town, unpublished paper.

Conner, S. and Kingman, S. (1989) *The Search for the Virus,* Penguin, London.

Conradie, D.P., Rabie, J. (1993) *Research amongst parents regarding HIV/AIDS and AIDS education programmes,* HSRC, unpublished.

Crewe, M. (1992) *AIDS in South Africa,* Penguin Forum Series, Johannesburg.

Cross, C. (1990) Africa and the people with no numbers: thoughts on outsider research, in Hugo, P., *Truth be in the Field,* pp. 24–44.

Cross, S. and Whiteside, A. (eds) (1993) *Facing up to AIDS: the socio-economic impact in southern Africa,* Macmillan, London.

Dauskardt, R. (1990) The changing geography of traditional

medicine; urban herbalism on the Witwatersrand, Johannesburg, *GeoJournal*, Vol. 22, No. 3, pp. 275–83.

——(1992) Of sickness and health: prospects for South African medical geography, in Rogerson, C. and McCarthy, J. (eds) *Geography in a changing South Africa – progress and prospects*, Oxford University Press, Cape Town, pp. 201–13.

Department of National Health and Population Development (1993) *Knowledge, attitudes, beliefs and sexual practices amongst persons with sexually transmitted infections with regard to sexuality and AIDS related issues*, Pretoria, unpublished.

Doyle, P. (1993) The demographic impact of AIDS on the South African population, in Cross, S. and Whiteside, A., *Facing up to AIDS*, pp. 87–112.

Duncan, C., Jones, K. and Moon, G. (1994) *Modelling the complexities of health related behaviour*, Annual Conference of the Institute of British Geographers, Nottingham, 1994.

Du Toit, B.M. (1987) Menarche and sexuality among a sample of black South African Schoolgirls, *Social Science and Medicine*, Vol. 24, No. 7, pp. 561–71.

Elmendorf, A.E. and Roseberry, W. (1993) Structural adjustment: what effect on health? On vulnerability to HIV? *AIDS Analysis Africa*, July/August 1993, pp. 4–7.

Epidemiological Comments (1994) Fourth national HIV survey of women attending antenatal clinics, South Africa, October/November 1993, Vol. 21, No. 4, pp. 68–79.

Everett, K. (1992) The development of an AIDS photo-comic for South African teenagers, *AIDS Bulletin*, Vol. 1, No. 2, pp. 7–9.

Evian, C. (1993) *Epidemiological patterns and the biological and socio-economic and political determinants of the spread of HIV infection in South Africa, and the implications for intervention programmes*, VIIIth International Conference on AIDS in Africa, Marrakesh, 1993.

Farmer, P. (1992) AIDS and anthropology in Haiti, in Herdt, G. and Lindbaum, S., *The Time of AIDS*, pp. 287–318.

Feldman, D. (1991) Comment of Packard, R. and Epstein, P. (1991) Epidemiologists, social scientists, and the structure of medical research on AIDS in Africa, *Social Science and Medicine*, Vol. 33, No. 7, pp. 771–94.

Feldman, D., O'Hara, P., Chitalu, N.W. and Lu, Y. (1995) *HIV prevention among Zambian adolescents: developing a value utilization/norm change model*, unpublished paper.

Finckenstein, B. (1990) AIDS in Namibia, in Stein, Z. and Zwi, A., *Action on AIDS in Southern Africa*, pp. 46–8.

Fisher, J.D. and Fisher, W.A. (1992) Changing high risk behaviour, *Psychological Bulletin*, Vol. 111, No. 3, pp. 455–74.

Fleming, A.F. (1992) South Africa and AIDS – seven years wasted, *Current AIDS Literature*, Vol. 5, No. 11, pp. 425–8.

——(1994a) To protect our children: a South African perspective, *AIDS Analysis Africa*, Vol. 4, No. 2, pp. 13–15.

——(1994b) A National AIDS Plan for South Africa, *AIDS Analysis Africa*, (Southern Africa Edition) Vol. 5, No. 2, pp. 9–11.

Fleming, A.F., Carballo, M., FitzSimons, D.W., Bailey, M.R. and Mann, J. (eds) (1988) *The Global Impact of AIDS*, Alan Liss Inc., New York.

Flint, J. (1994) Tanzania's AIDS truths, *WorldAIDS*, No. 33, p. 10.

Friedland, R.H. *et al.* (1991) Perception and knowledge about AIDS among students in university residences, *South African Medical Journal*, Vol. 79, pp. 754–57.

Fylkesnes, K., Brunborg, H. and Msiska, R. (1995) *An update on the current HIV/AIDS situation and future demographic impact*, paper presented at a conference on socio-economic impact of HIV/AIDS in Zambia, Lusaka, May 1995.

Gagnon, J. H. (1992) Epidemics and researchers: AIDS and the practice of social studies, in Herdt, G. and Lindenbaum, S., *The Time of AIDS*, pp. 27–40.

Giddens, A. (1984) *The Constitution of Society: Outline of the Theory of Structuration*, Polity Press, Cambridge.

Gottschalk, K. (1988) The political economy of health care: colonial Namibia 1915–1961, *Social Science and Medicine*, Vol. 26, No. 6, pp. 577–82.

Gould, P. (1993) *The Slow Plague*, Blackwell, London.

Govender, V., Bhana, R., Pillay, A. *et al.* (1992) Perceptions and knowledge about AIDS among family planning clinic attenders in Johannesburg, *South African Medical Journal*, Vol. 81, pp. 71–4.

Green, E.C., Zokwe, B., Dupree, J.D. (1995) The experience of an AIDS prevention program focused on South African traditional healers, *Social Science and Medicine*, Vol. 40, No. 4, pp. 503–15.

Gregson, S. and Foster, G. (1994) Modelling the spread of HIV-1 in Zimbabwe: Determinants, demographic impact and socio-economic consequences, *ZAINet AIDS News*, Vol. 2, No. 2, June 1994, pp. 2–7.

Guay, L., Hom, D., Mmiro, F. *et al.*, (1995) *Detection of HIV-1*

DNA and p24 antigen in breast milk and vertical transmission in Uganda, IXth International Conference on HIV/AIDS in Africa, Kampala, December 1995.

Hailonga, P. (1993) *A study to identify adolescents' knowledge, attitudes and belief towards teenage pregnancy*, Ministry of Health and Social Services, Windhoek, Namibia.

Hambridge, M. (1990) AIDS/HIV and Social Dislocation in Natal, *AIDS Analysis Africa* (Southern Africa edition), Vol. 1, No. 3, pp. 1–2.

——(1991) Migrant Labour and its impact on AIDS/HIV, *AIDS Analysis Africa* (Southern Africa edition), Vol. 2, No. 1, pp. 6–7.

Hamilton, R. (1991) *Special Issue on AIDS*, South African Institute of Race Relations Update 14, Johannesburg.

Haran, L. (1991) Tswana Medicine in interaction with Bio-medicine, *Social Science and Medicine*, Vol. 33, No. 2, pp. 167–75.

Hayes, M.V. (1992) On the epistemology of risk: language, logic and social science, *Social Science and Medicine*, Vol. 35, No. 4, pp. 401–7.

Head, J. (1992) *Transformation of the Structure of Poverty in the Struggle for an effective HIV/AIDS policy*, Paper presented at the Ruth First Memorial Colloquium, University of the Western Cape, August 1992.

Health Services Development Unit (1984) *Aspects of rural health services development; Experience from work in Mhala in the Eastern Transvaal, 1982–84*, HSDU, University of the Witwatersrand, Johannesburg.

Herdt, G. and Lindenbaum, S. (eds) (1992) *The Time of AIDS: Social Analysis, Theory, and Method*, Sage Publications, London.

Herod, A. (1993) Gender issues in the use of interviewing as a research method, *Professional Geographer*, Vol. 45, No. 3, pp. 305–15.

Heywood, M. (1996) Mining industry enters a new era of AIDS prevention, *AIDS Analysis Africa*, Vol. 6, No. 3, p. 16.

Holmshaw, A. (1992) When will they ever learn?, *Current AIDS Literature*, Vol. 5, No. 5, pp. 149–50.

Hu, D.J., Dondero, T.J., Rayfield, M.A. *et al.*, (1996) The emerging genetic diversity of HIV, *Journal of the American Medical Association*, Vol. 275, No. 3, pp. 210–16.

Hugo, P. (ed.) (1990) *Truth be in the Field: Social Science Research in Southern Africa*, University of South Africa Press, Pretoria.

IJsselmuiden, C.B., Padayachee, G.N., Mashaba, W. *et al.* (1990) Knowledge, beliefs and practices among black goldminers relating to the transmission of HIV and other sexually transmitted diseases, *South African Medical Journal*, Vol. 78, pp. 520–3.

Iranganyuma, B.M. (1993) *Socio-economic factors as a function of HIV/AIDS transmission among street children: the case study of HIV/AIDS risks among street children in Dar es Salaam, Tanzania*, VIIIth International Conference on AIDS in Africa, Marrakesh, 1993.

Jacobs, B., Miwe, J., Klokke, A.H. *et al.* (1993) *Secondary school students: a safer blood donor population in an urban settlement with high HIV prevalence in Africa*, VIIIth International Conference on AIDS in Africa, Marrakesh, 1993.

Jochelson, K., Mothibeli, M. and Leger, J.P. (1991) HIV and Migrant Labour in South Africa, *International Journal of Health Services*, Vol. 21, No. 1, pp. 157–70.

Kahenya, G. and Lake, S. (1995) *User fees and their impact on utilisation of key health services; summary report of a study carried out in Lusaka Urban 1994*, Ministry of Health, Government of Zambia, UNICEF.

Kaicener, J. (1993) *AIDS research among hostel dwellers*, Department of National Health and Population Development, unpublished.

Kapiga, S.H., Lwihula, G.K., Shao, J.F. *et al.* (1993) *Predictors of high risk sexual behaviour and condom use among women in Dar es Salaam, Tanzania*, VIIIth International Conference on AIDS in Africa, Marrakesh, 1993.

Karstaedt, A.S. (1992) AIDS – the Baragwanath experience. Part III. HIV infection in adults at Baragwanath Hospital, *South African Medical Journal*, Vol. 82, pp. 95–7.

Kasoma, F.P. (1994) *Content analysis of AIDS stories in the Zambian press*, Morehouse School of Medicine, unpublished, Lusaka.

Kato, S.P.W. (1993) *Role of economic independency in the fight against AIDS and STD*, VIIIth International Conference on AIDS in Africa, Marrakesh, 1993.

Kearns, R.A. and Joseph, A.E., (1993) Space in its place: developing the link in medical geography, *Social Science and Medicine*, Vol. 37, No. 6, pp. 711–17.

Kigaru, K., Krenn, S.C., Church, C. *et al.* (1993) *Gender differentials in AIDS awareness in Nigeria*, VIIIth International Conference on AIDS in Africa, Marrakesh, 1993.

Kiire, C.F. (1993) The epidemiology and control of Hepatitis B in sub-Saharan Africa, *Progress in Medical Virology*, Vol. 40, pp. 141–56.

Kleinman, A. (1978) Concepts and a model for the comparison of medical systems as cultural systems, *Social Science and Medicine*, Vol. 12, No. 1, pp. 85–93.

Klouda, A. (1992) Shifting patterns in international financing for AIDS programs, in Mann, J., *et al.*, *AIDS in the World*, pp. 787–801.

——(1994) It's called fiddling while Rome burns, *AIDS Analysis Africa*, Vol. 4, No. 3, pp. 9–11.

Konde-Lulu, J.K., Musagara, M. and Musgrave, S. (1993) Focus group interviews about AIDS in Rakai District in Uganda, *Social Science and Medicine*, Vol. 37, No. 5, pp. 679–84.

Kotze, J.C. (1992) *Children and the family in a rural settlement in Gazankulu*, Rand Afrikaans University, Johannesburg, unpublished.

Kronenfeld, J.J., Glik, D.C. and Jackson, K. (1993) Risk perceptions and AIDS, in Albrecht, G. and Zimmerman, R.S., *Advances in Medical Sociology, Volume 3: The social and behavioural aspects of AIDS*. JAI Press, London, pp. 37–57.

Laga, M., Nzila, N. and Goeman, J. (1991) The interrelationship of sexually transmitted diseases and HIV infection; implications for the control of both epidemics in Africa, in Piot, P. *et al.*, *AIDS in Africa*, pp. 55–63.

Lamptey, P., Coates, T., Slutkin, G. and Piot, P. (1993) HIV prevention – is it working? *AIDS Analysis Africa*, July/August 1993, pp. 2–3.

Leavitt, S.C. (1991) Sexual ideology and experience in a Papua New Guinea Society, *Social Science and Medicine*, Vol. 33, No. 8, pp. 897–907.

Lecatsas, G., Joubert, J.J., Schutte, C.H.J. *et al.*, (1989) *Peak prevalence of HIV in Namibian teenagers*, Vth International Conference on AIDS, Montreal, 1989.

Le Fanu, J., How potent males aid a killer virus, *Daily Telegraph*, 29 September 1991.

Lesetedi, L.T., Joubert, J.J., Schutte, C.H.J. et al. (1989) *Botswana Family Health Survey II, 1988*, place of publication unknown.

Linden, C., Allen, S., Carael, M. *et al.* (1991) Knowledge, attitudes, and perceived risk of AIDS among urban Rwandan women: relationship to HIV infection and behaviour change, *AIDS*, Vol. 5, pp. 993–1002.

Lindsay, J. (1989) Population control policies in Namibia, University of Leeds, *Southern African Studies*, No. 3, University of Leeds, Leeds.

Loslier, L. (1993) Ambiocontrol as a primary factor of health, *Social Science and Medicine*, Vol. 37, No. 6, pp. 735–43.

Lucas, S. (1992) *Interaction between AIDS programmes and development programmes*, VIIIth International Conference on AIDS, Amsterdam, 1992.

Manci, M. (1993) *Traditional medicine, practice in HIV/AIDS and sexually transmitted disease prevention in South Africa*, VIIIth International Conference on AIDS in Africa, Marrakesh, 1993.

Manderson, L. and Aaby, P. (1992) An epidemic in the field? Rapid assessment procedures and health research, *Social Science and Medicine*, Vol. 35, No. 7, pp. 839–50.

Mann, J., Tarantola, D.J.M. and Netter, T.W. (eds) (1992) *AIDS in the World*, Harvard University Press, Cambridge, MA and London.

Masters, W.H., Johnson, V.E. and Kolodny, R.C. (1988) *Crisis: Heterosexual Behaviour in the Age of AIDS*, Grafton, London.

Mathews, C., Kuhn, L., Metcalf, C.A., Joubert, G. and Cameron, N.A. (1990) Knowledge, attitudes and beliefs about AIDS in township school students in Cape Town, *South African Medical Journal*, Vol. 78, pp. 511–16.

Mattossovich, D., Caprara, D., Carrieri, M.P. *et al.* (1993) *Family dynamics and coping processes of AIDS patients in Abidjan, Côte d'Ivoire*, VIIIth International Conference on AIDS in Africa, Marrakesh, 1993.

May, R.M. and Anderson, R.M. (1987) Transmission dynamics of HIV infection, *Nature*, Vol. 326, pp. 137–42.

Mayer, J.D. (1983) The role of spatial analysis and geographic data in the detection of disease causation, *Social Science and Medicine*, Vol. 17, No. 16, pp. 1213–21.

——(1992) Challenges to understanding spatial patterns of disease: philosophical alternatives to logical positivism, *Social Science and Medicine*, Vol. 35, No. 4, pp. 579–87.

Mbizvo, M.T. and Adamchak, D.J. (1989) Condom use and acceptance: a survey of male Zimbabweans, *Central African Medical Journal*, Vol. 35, No. 11, pp. 519–23.

Mbizvo, M.T., Ray, S., Bassett, M. *et al.* (1993) *Condom use among urban, male factory workers in Harare, Zimbabwe*, VIIIth International Conference on AIDS in Africa, Marrakesh, 1993.

McIntyre, J.A. (1993) *Pregnancy and HIV infection at Baragwanath Hospital, 1987 to 1993*, VIIIth International Conference on AIDS in Africa, Marrakesh, 1993.

McMichael, A.J. (1993) *Planetary overload: Global environmental change and the health of the human species*, Cambridge University Press, Cambridge.

Mertens, T., Tondorf, G., Siebolds, M. *et al.* (1989) Epidemiology of HIV and Hepatitis B virus in selected African and Asian populations, *Infection*, Vol. 17, No. 1, pp. 4–7.

Mhloyi, G. and Mhloyi, M. (1990) *The Socio-cultural dimensions of AIDS in Zimbabwe*, VIth International Conference on AIDS, San Francisco.

Moodie, T.D. (1988) Migrancy and male sexuality on the South African gold mines, *Journal of Southern African Studies*, Vol. 14, No. 2, pp. 228–56.

Moses, S., Plummer, F.A., Bradley, J.E., Ndinya-Achola, J.O., Nagelkerke, J.D. *et al.* (1994) The association between lack of male circumcision and risk for HIV infection: a review of of the epidemiological data, *Sexually Transmitted Diseases*, Vol. 21, No. 4, pp. 201–10.

Mouli, C.V. (1992) *All against AIDS: the Copperbelt Health Education Project*, Zambia, Strategies for hope, No. 7, ActionAid, Amref, Christian Aid, London.

Msiska, R., Nangawe, E., Mulenga, D., Sichone, M., Kamanga, J. *et al.* (1995) *Factors determining health seeking behaviour patterns in Lusaka, Zambia – with particular relevance to sexually transmitted diseases*, Applied health research series report 1, National AIDS/STD/TB and Leprosy Programme, Ministry of Health, Lusaka.

Mulenga, C. (1993) *Orphans, widows and widowers in Zambia: a situation analysis and options for HIV/AIDS survival assistance*, Social Policy Research Group, University of Zambia/Ministry of Health, Lusaka.

Murphey, D. (1993) *The Ukimwi Road, from Kenya to Zimbabwe*, John Murray, London.

Musto, D.F. (1988) Quarantine and the problem of AIDS, in Fee, E. and Fox, D.M. (eds) *AIDS: the burdens of history*, University of California Press, Berkeley, CA and London, pp. 67–86.

Nagelkereke, N., Moses, S., Embree, F., Plummer, F. (1995) *The optimal duration of breastfeeding by HIV-1 infected mothers: balancing benefits*, IXth International Confernce on HIV/AIDS in Africa, Kampala, 1995.

Namibian Institute for Social and Economic Research (NISER) (1991) *Let's Crush AIDS: National AIDS Awareness Survey*, National AIDS Control Programme, University of Namibia, Windhoek.

National AIDS Convention of South Africa (NACOSA) (1992) *Report on the Conference of the National AIDS Convention of South Africa* (NACOSA), October, 1992, Sunnyside, Pretoria.

——(1994) *A National AIDS Plan for South Africa*, July 1994, Sunnyside, Pretoria.

Nduati, R., John, G.C., Richardson, B.A., *et al.* (1995) *HIV-1 infected cells in breastmilk: association with immunosuppression and vitamin A deficiency*, IXth International Conference on HIV/AIDS in Africa, Kampala, 1995.

Ntawuruhunga, J., Ladner, J., Malatre, X. *et al.* (1993) *Utilisation des préservatifs et impact du conseilling chez les femmes en âge de procreer. Une étude de cohorte à Kigali, Rwanda, 1992–1993*, VIIIth International Conference on AIDS in Africa, Marrakesh, 1993.

Nyamuryeking'e, K., Killewo, J., Hayes, R. *et al.* (1993) *Are routinely collected blood donor data useful for HIV surveillance in Africa?* VIIIth International Conference on AIDS in Africa, Marrakesh, 1993.

Nyudzewira, M., O'Dell, V., Waindim, P. *et al.* (1993) *Knowledge of AIDS/STDs, sexual practices and condom use in Limbe, Cameroon*, VIIIth International Conference on AIDS in Africa, Marrakesh, 1993.

O'Farrell, N., Hoosen, A.A., Coetzee, K.D. et al. (1991) Genital Ulcer Disease in women in Durban, South Africa, *Genitourinary Medicine*, Vol. 67, pp. 327–30.

O'Farrell, N. and Windsor, I. (1989) Enhanced transmission of HIV to women in South Africa, *British Medical Journal*, Vol. 298, pp. 1035.

Packard, R. (1989) *White Plague, Black Labor*, University of Natal Press, Pietermaritzburg.

——(1994) *White Plague, Black Labor Revisited: Tuberculosis in Contemporary South Africa*, Paper prepared for CRCSA Annual Workshop, Queen's University, Kingston, Ontario, January 1994.

Packard, R.M. and Epstein, P. (1991) Epidemiologists, social scientists, and the structure of medical research on AIDS in Africa, *Social Science and Medicine*, Vol. 33, No. 7, pp. 771–94.

Panos (1990) *Triple Jeopardy: Women and AIDS*, Panos Institute, London.

——(1992) *The Hidden Costs of AIDS: the challenge of HIV to development*, Panos Institute, London.

Parker, R.G., Herdt, G. and Carballo, M. (1991) Sexual culture, HIV transmission and AIDS research, *The Journal of Sex Research*, Vol. 28, No. 1, pp. 77–98.

Pendleton, W., LeBeau, D. and Tapscott, C. (1992) *Socio-economic study of the Ondangwa/Oshakati nexus area*, Namibian Institute for Social and Economic Research, University of Namibia, Windhoek.

Philips, D. (1990) *Health and Health Care in the Third World*, Longman, London.

Piot, P. (1993) *Public health sector strategies for the control of STDs today*, VIIIth International Conference on AIDS in Africa, Marrakesh, 1993.

Piot, P., Kapita, B.M. and Were, J.B.O. (eds) (1991) AIDS in Africa, *Current Science*, London.

Preston, R. (1993); *The integration of returned exiles, former combatants and other war-affected Namibians, Final Report*. Namibian Institute for Social and Economic Research, University of Namibia, Windhoek.

Preston-Whyte, E. and Zondi, M. (1989) To control their own reproduction: the agenda of black teenage mothers in Durban, *Agenda*, Vol. 4, pp. 47–67.

Radebe, M.B. (1991) *Research study on attitudes towards teenage pregnancy, Tintswalo Hospital*, Acornhoek, unpublished.

Richter, L. (1995) AIDS and South African street youth, *AIDSLINK*, No. 20, p. 8.

Robinson, J., Hayes, R., Mulder, D. and Auvert, B. (1993) *The proportion of HIV infections attributable to other STDs: simulation model estimates*, VIIIth International Conference on AIDS in Africa, Marrakesh, 1993.

Rossi, M.M. and Reijer, P. (1995) *Prevalence of orphans and their educational status in Nkwazi Compound – Ndola*, paper presented at the Vth Zambian National AIDS Conference, Lusaka, May 1995.

Roundy, R.W. (1987) Human behavioural disease hazards in Ethiopia; Spatial perspectives on rural health, in Akhtar, R. (ed) *Health and Disease in Tropical Africa: Geographical and Medical Viewpoints*, Harwood Academic, Yverdon, Switzerland.

Rowley, J., Anderson, R.M. and Ng, T.W. (1990) Reducing the spread of HIV infection in sub-Saharan Africa: some demographic and economic implications, *AIDS*, Vol. 4, pp. 47–56.

Russell, C. (1991) The AIDS crisis: a mining industry perspective, *Mining Survey*, No. 2, pp. 21–31.

Saayman, W. (1991) Some reflections on AIDS, ethics and the community in southern and central Africa, *Theologica Evangelica*, Vol. 24, No. 3, pp. 23–30.

Sabatier, R. (1988) *Blaming Others: prejudice, race and world-wide AIDS*, Panos Institute, London.

St. Francis' Hospital, Katete (1993) *HIV/AIDS Activities, 1993*, unpublished report, Katete, Zambia.

Sanders, D. and Abdulrahman, S. (1991) AIDS in Africa: the implications of economic recession and structural adjustment, *Health Policy and Planning*, Vol. 6, No. 2, pp. 157–65.

Saul, J.S. (1994) *Writing the Thirty Years' War for Southern African Liberation (1960–1990): What Criteria? What Narrative?* Journal of Southern African Studies Anniversary Conference, York, September 1994.

Saunders, R. (1991) Trucking around with death, *Africa South*, September 1991, pp. 38–9.

Schneider, H. and McIntyre, J. (1994) Is the 1993/4 AIDS Programme budget adequate? *South African Medical Journal*, Vol. 84, pp. 191–3.

Schoepf, B.G. (1991) Ethical, methodological and political issues of AIDS research in Central Africa, *Social Science and Medicine*, Vol. 33, No. 7, pp. 749–63.

——(1993) AIDS Action-research with women in Kinshasa, Zaire, *Social Science and Medicine*, Vol. 37, No. 11, pp. 1401–13.

Schopper, D., Doussantousse, S. and Orav, J. (1993) Sexual behaviour relevant to HIV transmission in a rural population. How much can a KAP survey tell us? *Social Science and Medicine*, Vol. 37, No. 3, pp. 401–12.

Schoub, B. (1992) AIDS in South Africa – into the next decade, *South African Medical Journal*, Vol. 81, pp. 55–6.

Schoub, B., Martin, D, Johnson, S. *et al.* (1989) *Development of the AIDS epidemic in South Africa*, Vth International Conference on AIDS, Montreal, 1989.

Seeley, J.A., Kengeya-Kayondo, J.F. and Mulder, D.W. (1992) Community-based HIV/AIDS research – whither community participation? Unsolved problems in a research programme in rural Uganda, *Social Science and Medicine*, Vol. 34, No. 10, pp. 1089–95.

Seidel, K., Eimbeck, A. and Goraseb, M. (1993a) *Safe transfusion is achievable; the Namibian experience in blood transfusion services*, VIIIth International Conference on AIDS in Africa, Marrakesh, 1993.

Seidel, K., Imbondi, S. and Lyambo, S. (1993b) *Selection criteria for blood donors with respect to HIV infection*, VIIIth International Conference on AIDS in Africa, Marrakesh, 1993.

Semba, R.D., Miotti, P.G., Chiphangwi, J.D. *et al.* (1994) Maternal vitamin A deficiency and mother to child transmission of HIV-1, *The Lancet* 1994, 343, pp 1593–7.

Serwadda, D., Wawer, M., Musgrave, S. *et al.* (1992) HIV risk factors in three geographic strata of rural Rakai District, Uganda, *AIDS*, Vol. 6, pp. 983–9.

Shannon, G. (1993) Communities, AIDS and Geography, *Social Science and Medicine*, Vol. 37, No. 5, pp. v–vii.

Shannon, G., Pyle, G.F. and Bashshur, R.L. (1991) *The Geography of AIDS: the origins and course of an epidemic*, Guilford Press, New York.

Sidaway, J.D. (1992) In other worlds: on the politics of research by 'First World' geographers in the 'Third World', *Area*, Vol. 24, No. 4, pp. 403–8.

Simenson, J.N., Plummer, F.A., Ngugi, E.N. *et al.* (1990) HIV infection among lower socio-economic strata prostitutes in Nairobi, *AIDS*, Vol. 4, pp. 139–44.

Simon, D. and Preston, R. (1993) Return to the promised land; the repatriation and resettlement of Namibian refugees, 1989–1990, in Black, R. and Robinson, V. (eds) (1993) *Geography and refugees; patterns and processes of change*, Belhaven, London.

Sitas, F., Fleming, A.F. and Morris, J. (1994) Residual risk of HIV transmission through blood transfusion in South Africa, *South African Medical Journal*, Vol. 84, pp. 142–4.

Skinner, D. (1992) *A review of studies of knowledge, attitudes, beliefs and behaviour in relation to HIV and AIDS within the South African context*, Association for Sociology in South Africa Conference, Pretoria, 1992.

Smallman-Raynor, M. and Cliff, A.D. (1992) Seasonality in Tropical AIDS: A geographical analysis, *International Journal of Epidemiology*, Vol. 21, No. 3, pp. 547–56.

Smallman-Raynor, M., Cliff, A. and Haggett, P. (1992) *Atlas of AIDS*, Blackwell, London.

Sokal, D.C., Buzingo, T., Nitunga, N., Kadende, P. and Standaert, B. (1993) Geographic and temporal stability of HIV seroprevalence among pregnant women in Bujumbura, Burundi, *AIDS*, Vol. 7, pp. 1481–4.

Southall, H. (1993) South African Trends and Projections of HIV infection, in Cross, S. and Whiteside, A., *Facing up to AIDS*, pp. 61–86.

Soyinka, F., Bamgbose, J. and Onayemi, O. (1993) *Sexual networking leading to sexually transmitted diseases and HIV risk among secondary school children in Nigeria*, VIIIth International Conference on AIDS in Africa, Marrakesh, 1993.

Stadler, J. (1993) Bridewealth and the deferral of marriage: towards an understanding of marriage payments in Timbavati, Gazankulu, *Africa Perspective*, December 1993, pp. 62–7.

Standing, H. (1992) AIDS: conceptual and methodological issues in researching sexual behaviour in sub-Saharan Africa, *Social Science and Medicine*, Vol. 34, No. 5, pp. 475–83.

Stein, Z. and Zwi, A. (eds) (1990) *Action on AIDS in Southern Africa*. Maputo Conference on Health in Transition in Southern Africa, April 1990, Committee for Health in Southern Africa, New York.

Stewart, J. (1993) *The impact of HIV/AIDS on the Health Sector in Natal/Kwazulu*, VIIIth International Conference on AIDS in Africa, Marrakesh, 1993.

Strachan, K. (1992) AIDS ignored by health department, say doctors, *Business Day*, 30 September 1992, p. 13.

Strebel, A. (1992) 'There's absolutely nothing I can do, just believe in God': South African women with AIDS, *Agenda*, July 1992, pp. 50–62.

Susser, M. (1987) *Epidemiology, health and society*. Oxford University Press, Oxford.

Tessier, S.F., Remy, G., Louis, J.P. and Trebucq, A. (1993) The frontline of HIV-1 diffusion in the Central African Region: A geographical and epidemiological perspective, *International Journal of Epidemiology*, Vol. 22, No. 1, pp. 127–33.

Treichler, P.A. (1992) AIDS, HIV, and the Cultural Construction of Reality, in Herdt, G. and Lindenbaum, S., *The Time of AIDS*, pp. 65–101.

Tshibangu, N.N. (1993) HIV infection in Boputhatswana; Epidemiologial surveillance 1987–1989, *South African Medical Journal*, Vol. 83, pp. 36–9.

Turshen, M. (1992) US Aid to AIDS in Africa, *Review of African Political Economy*, No. 55, pp. 95–101.

Turton, R.W. and Chalmers, B.E. (1990) Apartheid, stress and illness: the demographic context of distress reported by South Africans, *Social Science and Medicine*, Vol. 31, No. 11, pp. 1191–200.

Udvardy, M. (1988) Social and cultural dimensions for research on sexual behaviour related to HIV transmission: anthropological perspectives from Africa, in Sterky, G. and Krantz, I. (eds) *Society and HIV/AIDS*, Karolinka Institute, Department of International Health Care and Research, Stockholm, pp. 55–96.

Ulin, P.R. (1992) African women and AIDS: negotiating behavioural change, *Social Science and Medicine*, Vol. 34, No. 1, pp. 63–73.

UNDP (1993a) *Human Development Report 1993*, UNDP, Oxford University Press, Oxford.

——(1993b) *HIV and Development in Africa*, UNDP, Washington.

UNESCO and International Institute for Educational Planning (IIEP) (1993), *The impact of HIV/AIDS on education*, UNESCO, Paris.

UNICEF/Namibia (1990) *Report on a survey in Katutura and selected northern areas of Namibia in April–May, 1990*, UNICEF Namibia/Ministry of Health and Social Services, Windhoek.

UNICEF/Zimbabwe (1994) *Orphans and Children in Need: A Situation Analysis of Masvingo and Mwenezi Districts*, Department of Social Welfare, Harare.

Usher, A.D. (1992) After the Forest; AIDS as ecological collapse in Thailand, *Development Dialogue* Vol. 2, No. 1, pp. 13–49.

Van Aswegen, E. (1995) AIDS related knowledge – attitudes and behavioural practices among high school pupils, *South African Family Practice*, Vol 16, No. 5, May 1995, pp. 307–18.

Van Niftrik, J. (1992) The bumblers play on – a decade of debacle, *AIDS Analysis Africa* (Southern Africa edition), Vol. 3, No. 4, pp. 1–4.

——(1994) Women, adolescent and pre-adolescent, are at the leading edge of the HIV epidemic, *AIDS Analysis Africa*, Vol. 4, No. 2, pp. 11–12.

Vaughan, A. (1994) *Restructuring agricultural research in South Africa; meeting the needs of rural women, Journal of Southern African Studies* Anniversary Conference, York, September 1994.

Wakelin, P.M. (1983) *Migrant Labour in the Transkei, 1982*, Institute for Management and Development Studies, University of Transkei, Umtata.

Wallace, R. (1991) Social disintegration and the spread of

AIDS: thresholds for propagation along 'sociogeographic' networks, *Social Science and Medicine*, Vol. 33, No. 10, pp. 1155–62.

——(1993) Social disintegration and the spread of AIDS II; meltdown of sociogeographic structure in urban neighbourhoods, *Social Science and Medicine*, Vol. 37, No. 7, pp. 887–96.

Wardell, R. and Radebe, J. (1994) Counselling beyond the individual, *Positive Outlook*, Vol. 1, No. 3, p. 6.

Wawer, M.J., Serwadda, D., Musgrave, S.D. *et al.* (1991) Dynamics of spread of HIV-1 infection in a rural district of Uganda, *British Medical Journal*, Vol. 303, pp. 1303–6.

Webb, D. (1996a) *An Annotated Review of AIDS Research in Zambia*, NASTLP/UNICEF, Lusaka, 1996.

Webb, D. (1996b) Zambia's AIDS orphans will change the structure of society, *AIDS Analysis Africa*, June 1996, pp. 10–11.

Webb, D., Becci, M. and Bull, N. (1996) *The emergence of the adolescent in Zambia: the policy response challenge*, UNICEF Zambia, Lusaka 1996.

Webb, D. and Simon, D. (1993) *Migrants, money and the military; the social epidemiology of HIV/AIDS in Owambo, Northern Namibia*, Centre for Developing Areas Research, Research Papers No. 8, Royal Holloway, University of London.

West, M. (1990) Hostels, health and the nation, *South African Medical Journal*, Vol. 79, p. 691.

Whiteside, A. (1991) Urban demographic projections and AIDS, *Urban Forum*, Vol. 2, No. 1, pp. 107–12.

——(1993) *Socio-economic causes and consequences of HIV epidemic*, VIIIth International Conference on AIDS in Africa, Marrakesh, 1993.

——(1995) *Planning for AIDS Beyond the Social Sector*, IXth International Conference on AIDS in Africa, Kampala, 1995.

Williams, G. (1990) *From fear to hope; AIDS care and prevention at Chikankata Hospital, Zambia*, Strategies for Hope, No. 1, ActionAid, Amref, World in Need.

Williams, G. and Ray, S. (1993) *Work against AIDS; workplace-based AIDS initiatives in Zimbabwe*, Strategies for Hope, No. 8, ActionAid, Amref, London.

Willms, D. and Sewankambo, N.K. (1995) *An ethnographically derived model for eliciting and explaining socio-cultural determinants of risk for AIDS; 'risk realities, situations and events'*,

IXth International Conference on AIDS in Africa, Kampala, 1995.

Wilson, D., Greenspan, R. and Wilson, C. (1989) Knowledge about AIDS and self reported behaviour among Zimbabwean secondary school pupils, *Social Science and Medicine*, Vol. 28, No. 9, pp. 957–61.

Winn, S. and Skelton, R. (1992) HIV in the UK: Problems of prevalence, sociological response and health education, *Social Science and Medicine*, Vol. 34, No. 6, pp. 697–707.

World Bank (1993) *The economic impact of fatal adult illness in sub-Saharan Africa*, (workshop report), University of Dar es Salaam.

Yach, D. (1994) Health status and its determinants in South Africa, *Africa Health*, Special Supplement, March 1994, pp. 5–8.

Zambian Ministry of Health (1993) *National AIDS/STD/TB & Leprosy Programme; Behaviour change workshop, second medium term plan 1994–1998*, November 1993.

Zazayokwe, M. and Christie, G. (1990) *The role of traditional healers in combating AIDS in southern Africa*, VIth International Conference on AIDS, San Francisco.

Zimbabwe AIDS Network (ZAN)/Southern African AIDS Dissemination Service (1995) *Zimbabwe AIDS Directory – 1995*, Harare.

Zwi, A. and Bachmeyer, D. (1990) HIV and AIDS in South Africa: what is an appropriate public health response? *Health Policy and Planning*, Vol. 5, No. 4, pp. 316–26.

Zwi, A. and Cabral, A.J.R. (1991) Identifying 'high risk situations' for preventing AIDS, *British Medical Journal*, Vol. 303, pp. 1527–29.

Glossary and List of Acronyms and Abbreviations

aetiology, the cause(s) of a disease.
AIDS, Acquired Immune Deficiency Syndrome.
ANC, African National Congress.
anomie, feeling of anonymity and insecurity, usually in an urban setting.
APLA, Azanian People's Liberation Army.
ARC, AIDS-Related Complex.
ATICC, AIDS Training, Information and Counselling Centre.
CBO, Community-based organisation.
COSATU, Congress of South African Trade Unions.
cuca shop, a small informal bar (Owambo).
DHA, District Health Authority.
DNHPD, Department of National Health and Population Development.
ELISA, Enzyme-Linked Immuno-Sorbant Assay.
ESAP, Economic Structural Adjustment Programme.
GAPC, Global AIDS Policy Coalition.
GNU, Government of National Unity.
GPA, Global Programme on AIDS.
GUD, Genital Ulcer Disease.
hi hi, hypertension, high blood pressure.
HIV, Human Immuno-deficiency Virus.
HSDU, Health Services Development Unit, University of the Witwatersrand.
HSRC, Human Sciences Research Council.
HTLV, Human T-cell Lymphotropic Virus.
IFP, Inkatha Freedom Party.
IMF, International Monetary Fund.
induna, tribal councillor/headman.
Inhwalo, a payment of damages for pregnancy by the male or male's family amongst the Zulus.

inyanga, traditional herbalist. They often dispense herbs after the patient has consulted a diviner, or they prescribe herbs themselves.

IVDU, Intravenous Drug Use.

KAPB, Knowledge, Attitude, Practice and Belief survey.

lekgowa, white person (Northern Sotho).

lobola, bridewealth payment by the husband to the family of the bride. The payment was traditionally in the form of livestock, but increasingly the payment is in the form of cash. The value of the *lobola* varies according to individual cases, and is often decided upon externally, for example by the *induna*.

muti, traditional medicines/remedies.

NACOSA, National AIDS Convention of South Africa.

NACP, National AIDS Control Programme.

NANASO, Namibian Network of AIDS Service Organisations.

NAP, National AIDS Plan (South Africa).

NDF, Namibian Defence Force.

NGO, Non-Governmental Organisation.

NGU, Non-Gonococcal Urethritis.

NHA, National Health Authority.

NORAD, Norwegian Agency for Development

NUM, National Union of Mineworkers.

omahangu, variety of millet grown in northern Namibia (Owambo).

OPD, Out-Patients Department.

oshanas, small shallow depressions which flood during the rainy season, found in northern Namibia.

Owambo, former Namibian *bantustan* in the north of the country which is now divided into the regions of Omusati, Oshana, Ohangwena and Oshikoto. Owambo is also the umbrella term for the several ethnic groups of this area.

PAC, Pan Africanist Congress.

pandemic, disease prevalent across a whole country or the world.

parenteral infection, infection occurring through needlestick injury, or through the re-use of infected, unsterilised needles.

pathogen, agent causing disease.

PHA, Provincial Health Authority.

PHC, Primary Health Care.

phenomenology, approach (and philosophy) within the social sciences which explores the subjective nature of the environment and people's interaction with it, often through the examination of 'life worlds'.

PLAN, People's Liberation Army of Namibia.

PPHCN, Progressive Primary Health Care Network.

prevalence rate, the proportion of a defined group having a condition at one point in time.

PWA, Person with AIDS.

PWV, Pretoria, Witwatersrand Vereeniging nexus.

Rand, monetary unit of both South Africa and Namibia. During the period of field work the exchange rate was approximately R5 = £1. From September 1993 the Namibia Dollar was introduced in parallel with the Rand, with which it is fully convertible at parity.

RAP, Rapid Assessment Procedures.

RDP, Reconstruction and Development Programme.

retrovirus, any of a group of RNA viruses which form DNA during the replication of their RNA. HTLV and HIV are examples of retroviruses.

RWA, Relative with AIDS.

SACP, South African Communist Party.

SADF, South African Defence Force.

SAFO, Society for AIDS Families and Orphans (Soweto).

SANASO, Southern African Network of AIDS Service Organisations.

sangoma, traditional healer/diviner. Trained to identify the 'sorcerer' and is usually a woman. They 'throw the bones' and consult the ancestors in order to identify the causes of sickness and appropriate prescriptions. Deals in animal matter as well as herbal remedies.

SAP, Structural Adjustment Policy.

sefebe, Northern Sotho word meaning 'loose'/sexually promiscuous woman.

shebeen, informal (and previously illicit) bar.

SIDA, Swedish International Development Authority.

SIV, Simian Immuno-deficiency Virus.

spaza, small informal shop, selling food and everyday goods.

STD, Sexually Transmitted Disease.

stokvel, community-based rotating credit scheme.

SWAPO, South West Africa People's Organisation.

TASO, The Aids Service Organisation.

TB, Tuberculosis.

TGWU, Transport and General Workers' Union.

Tsonga, ethnic group of the eastern Transvaal, inhabiting the Mapulaneng area of former Lebowa.

ukujami, traditional thigh sex (Swazi).

ukusoma, traditional thigh sex (Zulu).

UN, United Nations.

UNAIDS, Joint United Nations Programme on HIV/AIDS.

UNDP, United Nations Development Programme.

UNESCO, United Nations Educational, Scientific and Cultural Organisation.

UNFPA, United Nations Population Fund

UNICEF, United Nations Children's Fund.

UNTAG, United Nations Transitional Assistance Group.

USAID, United States Agency for International Development.

veld, Afrikaans word meaning 'open grass country'.

WHO, World Health Organization.

Wits, University of the Witwatersrand, Johannesburg.

Witwatersrand/'Rand', ('White water's ridge') Afrikaans word for the area surrounding Johannesburg, corresponding to the area of gold deposits.

ZINATHA, Zimbabwean National Association of Traditional Healers.

Index

Printed and bound by CPI Group (UK) Ltd, Croydon, CR0 4YY

09/06/2025